WEEDING OUT
WHEAT

A SIMPLE, SCIENTIFIC,
FAITH-BASED GUIDE

BY LUKE & TRISHA
GILKERSON

Disclaimer:
Information shared in this ebook is from our own research, experience, and opinion. We are not medical professionals. This is for informational and entertainment purposes only and to be used only with the clearance of your own medical professional.

Contact Luke and Trisha via email at IntoxicatedOnLifeMail@ gmail.com.

COMING EARLY IN 2014:

Deciding to go wheat-free can be a pretty big challenge. To help you with your journey, we are putting together a cookbook with some of our favorite wheat-free recipes.

Sign up to receive your complimentary copy at *IntoxicatedOnLife.com/WOWcookbook*

TABLE OF CONTENTS

FOREWORD

BY: JIMMY MOORE

It's nearly impossible to ignore the significant health decline we have been experiencing over the past few decades. Obesity, heart disease, and diabetes have been allowed to skyrocket to epidemic proportions unlike anything we have ever seen in the history of the world.

All of the so-called health "experts" almost universally point to a lack of physical activity and the overconsumption of dietary fat and calories, but what if that conventional thinking on nutrition as it relates to our health is missing a very critical element in the equation? Here's the million dollar question—what if people are being told to eat *more* of something that is the very culprit in bringing about the chronic weight and health issues that have collectively plagued us for so long?

This is the sordid tale about the "healthy whole grains" myth that Luke and Trisha Gilkerson do a fantastic job unraveling in this book.

THE CHRISTIAN PERSPECTIVE

With the enormous popularity of *New York Times* runaway bestselling books like *Wheat Belly* by cardiologist Dr. William Davis and *Grain Brain* by neurologist Dr. David Perlmutter, there is definitely an intense hunger and desire for more knowledge out there about the damaging impact that wheat is having on our health.

The unique aspect that Luke and Trisha have added to the conversation is how Christians should grapple with this knowledge about wheat-based foods like bread when it is talked about so frequently throughout the Bible. I get this very important question a lot from my blog readers: if this is supposed to be something that is so *bad* for our health, then why did the Lord use it so prominently in Biblical teachings and parables?

As a Christian who asked Jesus into my heart at the age of seven, I grew up reciting the Lord's Prayer that states "give us this day our daily bread." We also regularly participated in the holy act of communion that included a wafer made from wheat. All this bread imagery as a part of church culture may make some people of faith scoff at the idea that eating a wheat-free diet is something that would be pleasing to God? That's why this book is so critically important: to state clearly what the Bible actually says about wheat and bread, what the application of the commands are regarding those things, and how we can honor God by embracing a wheat-free lifestyle.

I've got to be 100% honest with you about something that is quite troubling to me as a Christian. While the body of Christ should be leading the way as an example of what healthy living looks like, the exact opposite is true. Some of the most overweight and unhealthy people in the world are Christians who may not even realize the negative impact that wheat is causing to the temple of the Holy Spirit.

Think about all the prayer requests that have been offered up for people dealing with their weight, diabetes, cancer, heart problems, and more. This book could be the answer to all those heartfelt prayers that have been lifted up over the years.

WITH GOD ALL THINGS ARE POSSIBLE

We can do a whole lot more work for the cause of Christ by living longer, healthier lives the wheat-free way, and *Weeding Out Wheat* shines a bright light on how to make that happen. Let this book guide you towards a practical, prudent path to physical and even spiritual healing.

In 2004, I weighed in at 410 pounds and was, by the grace of God, able to bring my weight down to 230 while restoring my health by eliminating grains, sugar, and starch from my diet. To say my life changed would be an understatement, and it goes well beyond the physical changes that are obvious. My relationship with the Lord, my wife, and my friends and family were all enhanced because I chose to make better decisions about my health. Today I try to be an example to other Christians about how they can make this miracle happen in their own lives. Remember the words of Jesus in Matthew 19:26 when he said "with man this is impossible, but with God all things are possible." This is our call to action, and I encourage you to pray earnestly that God would open your eyes of your need to do this.

I'm incredibly grateful to Luke and Trisha Gilkerson for having the courage and conviction to write this critical book that's needed now more than ever before, and I hope and pray that it blesses you with invaluable information that will enhance our witness for many years to come.

Jimmy Moore
"Livin' La Vida Low-Carb"
www.livinlavidalowcarb.com

WHEAT CAUSING A HEALTH CRISIS?
YEAH, RIGHT.

We get it. The idea of giving up your favorite breads and pastas sounds like complete madness. Trust us. We know. To this day, every time we drive by our old favorite Italian restaurant, we feel a sort of aching homesickness (mild exaggeration).

This book makes some unbelievable claims. You'll read about how wheat is most likely a common culprit contributing to digestive problems, asthma, irritable bowel syndrome, migraines, PMS, arthritis, Multiple Sclerosis (MS), infertility, miscarriages, heart disease, cancer, diabetes, anxiety, depression, autism, hyperactivity, schizophrenia, Attention Deficit Disorder (ADD), Attention Deficit Hyperactivity Disorder (ADHD), weight gain, sleep disturbances, nutritional deficiencies, and tooth decay. Totally outlandish, right?

The first time we started reading about this impressive list of health concerns, we simply couldn't wrap our minds around it.

"Come on," we said. "This is ridiculous. Wheat is a staple of life. It has been consumed by people for ages. How could something so fundamental to human culture and civilization be *that* bad for you?"

Furthermore, as Christians, we had a very hard time believing that something so central to the daily life of God's people throughout the Bible could be so poisonous. Didn't Jesus ask us to pray for "our daily bread"? Isn't He the "Bread of Life"? Don't we partake of the bread of Jesus' body when we gather for communion?

SEND IN THE NERDS

You probably know someone who has given up wheat or gone gluten-free. We know quite a few people who have—family, friends, and online acquaintances. Is it a fad? Or is there truly something to this?

The more we heard about wheat-free living, the more questions we had, so our nerdy brains went to work. I (Trisha) love reading medical journals. I (Luke) love the study of history and theology. Together, we decided to unleash the raw power of our nerdy brains and study this "fad."

If we were going to go wheat-free, we were going to do it like a boss.

Countless hours were spent reading articles, listening to lectures by physicians and researchers, and reading medical journals before we determined to take the wheat-free plunge. We hope you can benefit from the studying and reading we've done.

Our hope is to unpack some of the mystery, questions, and complicated research into a brief, understandable book so you can make the decision for yourself whether this is also a journey that is right for you and your family.

Along with that, we aim to give you some practical how-to's to get you started on your wheat-free journey.

And above all, we want to honor God with what we do, including what we put into our bodies. So, as with all of our decisions, the decision to go wheat-free was a spiritual decision as well. As Moses said, "Man does not live on bread alone"—in our case, we don't live on bread at all.

A FEW CAVEATS

With that said, we would like to note that we are not health care workers, and this is not an exhaustive review of the literature. We've done our best to communicate the science as best as we understand it, but there are much more qualified individuals out there who have written more detailed books on this topic.

While there are more comprehensive and scientifically detailed books, we hope this book will be an easy and accessible read for the lay-person.

We'd also like to note that we don't believe that wheat is the *only* cause of the plethora of modern diseases on the rise today. We don't think that giving up wheat is the panacea of perfect health. We *do* believe that wheat is one of the major players, but not the only player. We also believe the over-consumption of sugar is a major problem, consumption of genetically modified plants, produce that is laden in pesticides and chemicals, meat that has been pumped full of chemicals and raised in feed-lots, and the list goes on and on. But, you won't see us talking about those things in this book. This book is focused on the problems with wheat.

OUR JOURNEY, NOT YOURS

Ultimately, this research summarizes the information we read that led us to make the decision to go wheat-free. This may or may not be the path you take, and perhaps you will come to different conclusions than we did. We understand that the information in this book will not be the last word on the subject for you. Either way, we hope the information here is a good "first word" in your journey to better health.

TESTIMONIAL

"after I stopped eating wheat, the stomach aches were gone!"

Over two years ago I took the plunge and gave up wheat... and have never regretted that decision! For years I struggled with stomach aches and bloating after I ate. It got to the point where I dreaded eating because I knew I would not feel well afterward. It finally clicked that possibly wheat was the culprit. Sure enough, after I stopped eating wheat, the stomach aches were gone! I am so thankful for all of the people out there who educate and inform about wheat sensitivities. Without them (and the wonderful recipes they post!) I would have been lost. Now every time I accidentally eat something with wheat I know right away. I get symptoms similar to food poisoning. That is enough to keep me away from wheat for good!

—Erin from wateronthefloor.wordpress.com

OH, HOW TIMES HAVE CHANGED:

YESTERDAY'S WHEAT
VS.
TODAY'S WHEAT

A life without wheat makes about as much sense as a world without gravity. Wheat is not only a staple of modern American life, it has also been cultivated for centuries and is a part of the culinary heritage of many cultures. Giving up wheat, for many people, can feel like giving up a part of who they are.

Cultivating and breeding grain, as opposed to harvesting it from the wild, has been a practice in human cultures for thousands of years. The ability to cultivate wheat and other grains was a major turning point in human civilization, enabling more permanent settlements and thereby promoting human ingenuity and culture.

Our goal in this chapter is not to take you back before the days of wheat cultivation—though that is an interesting area of study—but rather to take you back just a few decades when modern wheat started to undergo major changes.

Cultivating grain has always involved a process of breeding in order to produce the best yield, but in the latter part of the twentieth century, this practice took on a whole new meaning. The wheat our great-grandparents ate is not the same as the wheat we eat today.

ANCIENT WHEAT

Einkorn wheat was among the first wild wheat grains cultivated by humans. Shortly after this, emmer, an offspring of einkorn and goatgrass, started to be grown in the Middle East.[1] This was most likely the wheat used by Israelites in the days of Moses and up through the age of the Greeks.

At the same time emmer naturally mixed with *Triticum tauschii,* creating *Triticum aestivum* (bread wheat), and this family of wheat was grown through the twentieth century. You can still find wild einkorn and emmer wheat today, found in small quantities scattered throughout the Middle East and southern Europe.

MODERN WHEAT

As industrialized farming became the norm, farmers wanted wheat that would be resistant to heat, disease, and drought, as well as wheat that would produce the greatest yield. The 1940's and 50's saw many innovations.

By the late 40's, researchers knew they could create huge yields of grain by applying nitrogen-rich chemical fertilizers to the wheat, but the heads of grain would become too large to be supported by the long stalks. So in the early 50's, Dr. Norman Borlaug, the director of the International Wheat Improvement Program, funded by the Rockefeller and Ford Foundations, discovered a way to breed semi-dwarf wheat stalks that wouldn't buckle under the weight of large seed heads. Dr. Borlaug's plants produced enormous heads of grain supported by sturdy stalks, tripling or quadrupling the amount of wheat an acre of land could produce.

For his work on increasing food production, Dr. Borlaug was awarded the Nobel Peace Prize in 1970. Upon his death a few years ago, the *New York Times* said Dr. Borlaug "did more than anyone else in the 20th century to teach the world to feed itself."[2] His work is credited with saving hundreds of millions of lives.

The Wall Street Journal said the day after his death, "more than any other single person Borlaug showed that nature is no match for human ingenuity in setting the real limits to growth."[3]

Of course, the desire to solve the world hunger problem is commendable, but it was assumed by scientists that modern wheat hybrids would offer humans the same nutritional value as before. Unfortunately, this is not the case. It is possible that this lack of testing ended up creating as many problems as it solved.

GLUTENSTEIN'S MONSTER

Only in recent years has there been pressure to test the impact of modern hybridization on human health. In the early decades, testing was not done because scientists assumed all hybridization was safe. But the hybridization methods we're talking here about aren't the changes we see occurring in nature.

Human beings have found a number of ways to change plants in recent years. Genetic modification is one such way. Genetic modification is inserting genes from one species into that of another species. Animal, bacteria, or virus genes can be inserted into plant DNA. Yes, this sounds like something out of a sci-fi movie, but it's real, and it's happening with our food. Studies are now showing, for instance, that when animals are fed genetically modified soybeans that are Roundup resistant, this alters their liver, pancreatic, intestinal, and testicular tissue. It is believed that these genetically altered foods now contain proteins that are toxic.[4]

Now, wheat is *not* (as of this printing) genetically modified like Roundup resistant soybeans, but the reason we draw this comparison is because many did not question the safety of these genetically modified plants until recently. So too, many are not questioning the safety of the mutant wheat we are consuming.

Though wheat has not been genetically modified, it has undergone something much more dangerous than the simple hybridization that Gregor Mendel, the father of modern genetics, demonstrated in pea plants. Wheat has undergone what is known as *transgenic breeding*.

Transgenic breeding is breeding of wheat embryos in the presence of radiation and/or harsh chemicals. Transgenic breeding may in fact be *more* dangerous than genetic modification of plants, and it appears there are no regulations at all on transgenic breeding. (More on this on the next page.)

"modern wheat has many more gluten proteins, which are associated with today's gluten sensitivities, such as celiac disease."

Scientists can compare the proteins found in wheat hybrids created from two parent strains. Gluten, one of the proteins in wheat, undergoes the greatest change. One experiment found fourteen *new* gluten proteins in the offspring that were not found in parent wheat plants.[5] When compared with wheat strains that are centuries old, modern wheat has many more gluten proteins, which are associated with today's gluten sensitivities, such as celiac disease.[6]

TEENAGE MUTANT NINJA WHEAT

Modern wheat has been so modified by humans, these strains are actually *unable* to grow in the wild anymore because they depend on pest control and nitrate fertilization.[7] (To use an analogy used by some doctors, what if you had a species of dog that was bred in such a way it couldn't survive in the wild anymore because it *had* to eat Purina Puppy Chow®?)

Indeed, most of the wheat produced today uses some type of pesticide. Of the 16 pesticides used on wheat, the most common type of pesticide used is Malathion, which is used on nearly 50% of all wheat. Malathion is a neurotoxin and classified as an "endocrine disruptor," meaning it can screw up the hormones in our bodies.[8]

As we've already mentioned, wheat seeds have been exposed to radiation.[9, 10, 11] When food-stuffs are subjected to high dose irradiation, the molecular structure of the food is changed, potentially creating carcinogens and toxic chemicals, and causing infertility, kidney damage, and changes the nutritional value of food.[12] This irradiation with the use of gamma and microwave rays has a number of doctors and scientists quite alarmed, and for good reason. Animal studies have resulted in some quite catastrophic outcomes.[13, 14, 15] These doctors and scientists have petitioned the government to halt irradiation of food, but have been met with deaf ears.[16]

THE SUGAR BUZZ OF DWARF WHEAT

As hybridization has increased, the mineral content of harvested wheat grains has also decreased. The Broadbalk Winter Wheat Experiment found that due to shorter stalks, less sun, and shallower roots systems, the common dwarf wheat is deficient in many vitamins and minerals.[17] Modern wheat is lower in minerals like zinc, magnesium, iron, copper, and selenium than its ancient ancestor.[18, 19]

Another difference we see is in how grains are being processed. Of course most grains are stripped of their bran and germ. But grains today are also ground much more finely than they were in ancient times. The grains are ground so finely that our body converts them to sugar much more quickly which leads to weight gain and a plethora of other problems.

Unfortunately, the impact of modern wheat has not been studied thoroughly, but the potential health concerns are great.

CAUSE FOR ALARM: WHEAT-ASSOCIATED PROBLEMS ON THE RISE

Could these modern wheat changes be one of the causes behind a rise in specific health problems today?

A 2009 study published in *Gastroenterology* compared 10,000 blood samples from Air Force recruits 50 years ago to 10,000 current samples. They were startled by the results. In just 50 years, there has been a *400% increase* in the prevalence of celiac disease.[20]

Celiac disease is when one of the wheat proteins—gluten—attacks the small intestine. This autoimmune disease causes inflammation and has the potential to cause a wide range of problems. The symptoms most commonly associated with celiac disease are diarrhea, cramping, and bloating, but there are a host of other problems. In fact, only a third of individuals with celiac disease experience any intestinal discomfort.

Celiac disease is just *one* type of sensitivity to wheat. Gluten allergies and sensitivities are also on the rise and are estimated to occur in approximately 18 million or more individuals in the U.S. alone. Gastroenterologist Dr. Richard Auld says ten years ago he would have thought the trend towards wheat-free living was just a fad, but now he thinks differently. "Gluten allergy—autoimmune disease—is much more common now than 50 years ago," he claims.[21]

Type 1 diabetes has also been rising sharply over the past several decades.[22] Lab experiments with mice show a strong connection between a wheat-fed diet and type 1 diabetes.[23]

CONNECTING THE DOTS

Unfortunately, it's quite difficult to determine who has a serious problem with wheat because the symptoms are so diverse and often doctors haven't been trained to associate the symptoms with wheat.

Certainly, not all our health problems are traced back to wheat. Far from it. But with the recent changes in our wheat crops, could the rise of wheat-related diseases be a consequence?

Thankfully, the tide seems to be turning. Doctors are being educated and some are beginning to connect the dots. They are realizing that, in fact, many of their patients do have a problem with wheat even if the "classic symptoms" of celiac disease are not present.

As a family, we started reading more and more about the scores of people who feel *dramatically* better after going wheat-free. Doctor after doctor tells their patients they can find nothing wrong with them, despite their chronic symptoms. But take away the wheat and the symptoms seem to stop.

The anecdotal evidence seems to be piling up.

TESTIMONIAL

"I took wheat out of my diet and my horrid health problems cleared up."

Gluten and I have had a long standing love/hate relationship. It all started a number of years ago when I was starting on my whole food journey. Naturally, I added in whole grain wheat to my diet.

And plenty of it.

Whole wheat pasta, whole grain bread, and more.

I remember walking down the street in my city after sampling some whole wheat bread. It tasted great, but I didn't feel so great. In fact, I felt horrid. Like I had been drugged.

The feeling came and went over the next few weeks. I was frightened and depressed. Eventually, I put 2 and 2 together and figured out it was likely wheat that was causing my issues.

I took wheat out of my diet and my horrid health problems cleared up.

As time went on, I added wheat back into my diet. Maybe I wasn't eating as much, but I didn't have that horrid feeling again.

Until many years later.

Since that time I have been through many things health-wise, but one recent occurrence has to do with wheat. For the most part, I have been gluten-free for the past few years.

We have very little gluten in our home, but when I go to Costco I will allow myself to sample some of their pastas and such.

Recently, I had some disconcerting thyroid issues. Some of my labs were abnormal, one of which was a thyroid antibody test. Not very abnormal, but elevated. In fact, one M.D. said I for sure didn't have an autoimmune issue, that is how "non elevated" they were.

However, I wasn't thrilled.

I scoured the internet and found that gluten is highly implicated in thyroid issues.

So completely off of gluten I went.

No Costco. Nothing.

Just the other day I got more blood work back. My antibody levels? They went down by almost 50% of the original elevation. Was it all because of my going completely sans gluten? I don't know, but I am not going back on.

—Adrienne from WholeNewMom.com

WHEAT GONE WILD:

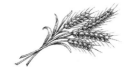

UNDERSTANDING WHEAT'S CONNECTION TO DETERIORATING HEALTH

SOME NECESSARY DEFINITIONS:

CELIAC DISEASE,
WHEAT ALLERGIES,
GLUTEN INTOLERANCE,
& GLUTEN SENSITIVITY

Before getting too far, it's necessary to give some explanation about some of the terminology you'll read, both in this book as well as in other books and medical journals.

In health literature, you'll probably come across some of these terms: celiac disease, gluten intolerance, gluten sensitivity, gluten syndrome, and gluten/wheat allergy. The terms that different people throw around can mean different things, and there is not complete consensus on what they should mean. They're often used interchangeably. Below are some guides on what these terms likely mean as you run across them.

WHEAT ALLERGIES

Gluten or wheat allergies refer to a response in the immune system. Any time someone is using the word "allergy," they are referring to your immune system over-reacting to something.

The immune system views the protein from the wheat as an invader and goes into attack mode—hence, you end up feeling miserable, at least to some extent. This acute reaction causes inflammation of various tissues and organs in the body. This inflammation leads to all sorts of internal damage to cells and tissues.

The problem with a wheat allergy is *you don't always know you have it.* Do you have repeated headaches, maybe migraines? PMS? Chronic sniffling or coughing? (More about these in the next chapter.) These are just a few examples of symptoms of a wheat allergy. Because wheat is such a prevalent staple in modern diets, many have a difficult time associating symptoms with wheat consumption.

GLUTEN INTOLERANCE

Gluten *intolerance* is not born in the immune system but is an inability to tolerate gluten in various tissues of the body, often the gut.

More times than not, those with a gluten intolerance are people whose bodies overproduce zonulin when they eat gluten. Too much zonulin in the system creates a "leaky gut," leading to an array of problems. Partially digested food from your gut leaks into the bloodstream, leading to a number of different food allergies. (These are *acquired* allergies—allergies to foods that people don't typically get until later in life.)

The problems don't stop with just allergies. As you can imagine, having poop in your bloodstream isn't going to do your body any favors.

GLUTEN SENSITIVITY AND CELIAC DISEASE

Gluten sensitivity or gluten-syndrome don't have specific definitions. They are used differently by different researchers and doctors, so the definitions are hard to nail down. These are often used as a mesh of the two above conditions (gluten allergies and gluten intolerance).

Gluten sensitivity is *not* the same as celiac disease, but gluten sensitivity can *cause* celiac disease.

Many people believe falsely that when people are sensitive to gluten, that must mean they have celiac disease. They think celiac disease is the *only* manifestation of having a problem with gluten. They make the incorrect assumption that if they don't have tummy issues, they should be fine.

Nothing could be farther than the truth. Celiac disease is only one evidence of gluten sensitivity. In fact, gluten sensitivity takes many, many forms. Often people who suffer from gluten sensitivity have no abdominal discomfort whatsoever.

Often the symptoms of gluten sensitivity go undetected and unnoticed for many years because they are not severe enough to interrupt people's lives.

People don't worry about the occasional migraine because everyone gets a headache now and then.

Stiff joints—just getting older.

PMS is normal, right?

Coughing and sniffles—just environmental allergies, I'm sure.

Gluten sensitivity often doesn't cause major interruption until it has attacked your body to the point that you must wake up and pay attention. Maybe the development of an autoimmune disease. Repeated miscarriages. Infertility.

The problem is, often people don't link these things to a problem with wheat, and your body can't heal from these diseases overnight. In fact, if the damage is too complete, your body may never fully heal.

Moral of the story: different people have different symptoms to wheat/gluten sensitivity. Pay attention to your body.

TESTIMONIAL

"I can't say enough about the benefits we experienced after taking out wheat."

My children began to have serious digestive problems after a year of massive exposure to toxic mold. After we left the home we began to revamp our diet. Two of the kids had elevated gliadin levels. We decided to take out wheat and eventually all grains. Our son with Type 1 diabetes and the horrible abdominal pain finally found relief for the discomfort. Another daughter with serious digestive pain noticed great improvement. I can't say enough about the benefits we experienced after taking out wheat.

—Andrea Fabry from www.It-Takes-Time.com/

IS WHEAT-FREE RIGHT FOR YOU?

INDICATIONS THAT YOU SHOULD CONSIDER A WHEAT-FREE DIET

Should you try a wheat-free diet? In short, *yes*. You should at least *try* a wheat-free diet. Given the serious problems with wheat that are on the rise, at a minimum, anyone living in this era should at least consider it.

In the next chapter you'll learn more about the *why*—why is wheat a less-than-ideal food? In this chapter, you will learn about the *what*—what medical conditions have been linked to wheat consumption?

The New England Journal of Medicine[24] reported there are 55 diseases that could potentially be caused by eating gluten, one of the proteins found in wheat. Other authors[25] have expanded this list to more than 200 conditions.

The conditions below represent a "short list."

Do you or close blood-relatives have any of these conditions?

DIGESTIVE PROBLEMS

Gastrointestinal problems are the classic marker of celiac disease and gluten intolerance. Symptoms can include bloating, cramping, diarrhea, constipation, irritable bowel syndrome, and indigestion. Contrary to popular opinion, these symptoms can also occur in non-celiac individuals—those who are just sensitive to wheat.[26]

However, it is important to note, the vast majority of people who have problems with wheat *don't* have noticeable stomach problems. Their problem with gluten is manifested in other ways.

MIGRAINES

With more than 10 million Americans who suffer from migraine headaches and billions of dollars in health care costs being spent because of them, migraines are kind of a big deal.[27] If you've never experienced one, migraines are like the Mac Daddy of all headaches. Seriously. They can cause not only your head to throb but also nausea, vomiting, and light sensitivity.

There are a number of triggers for migraines, food and chemical triggers being towards the top of the list. And, as you've probably already guessed, headaches, particularly migraines, are very commonly associated with gluten intolerance.[28, 29, 30, 31, 32]

When people get rid of the wheat and other trigger foods and focus on healing their gut, they often find their migraines subside.

PMS

Listen up, ladies. Are you ready to ditch the wild roller coaster ride of emotions each month? Though everyone says PMS is "normal" and just something you have to live with, it is not. PMS is certainly prevalent, but it should not ever be considered the norm.

Wheat can wreak havoc on a woman's hormonal balance. It's not just wheat that is to blame, of course; other classic offenders including soy and sugar can create problems as well. These foods are all highly inflammatory and, in addition, can cause digestive issues. The more foods you eat that disrupt the nourishment of your body, including your endocrine system (the thyroid gland, adrenals, pituitary gland, etc.) the crazier your roller coaster ride will be through your cycle. Many women find that simply giving up wheat and all gluten-containing products rectifies many of these hormonal imbalances, but being diligent to avoid other nasty foods like soy and sugar is a good idea, too.

INFERTILITY AND MISCARRIAGES

Gluten intolerance is often overlooked in couples suffering from infertility. A number of studies have linked infertility in both men and women—particularly those couples where no other explanation for infertility can be found.[33, 34, 35, 36, 37, 38, 39, 40, 41]

Likewise, women who have experienced multiple unexplained miscarriages should consider whether their consumption of wheat it playing a role. Just as wheat can cause hormonal problems that lead to infertility and PMS, so, too, can wheat cause problems with carrying a baby to term.[42, 43, 44, 45]

MOOD DISORDERS

Mood disorders like anxiety or depression have been also linked with gluten intolerance.[46, 47, 48] If you have long-standing mental health problems you may not have ever considered that a food could be causing all of the problems you're experiencing. Why not? A food like wheat, so prevalent and eaten in such abundance, could most certainly be causing or contributing to your anxiety or depression.

CHILDHOOD BRAIN DISORDERS

Childhood problems like learning disorders, autism, and hyperactivity can be caused by an intolerance to the proteins found in wheat. When the proteins in wheat cross into the brain, this is trouble. It is interesting to note that, children with autism spectrum disorders and those with ADD often see improvement when eliminating wheat from their diets.[49, 50, 51, 52, 53, 54, 55]

ASTHMA

Asthma can frequently be caused by food allergies, and a wheat allergy is one that often causes wheezing and chest discomfort in children and adults alike.[56, 57]

AUTOIMMUNE DISEASES

Along with celiac disease, which is the most commonly known autoimmune disease associated with gluten consumption. Autoimmune diseases such as arthritis,[58] autoimmune thyroid disorders,[59, 60, 61, 62, 63, 64, 65, 66, 67, 68, 69, 70, 71, 72] multiple sclerosis,[73] and more,[74, 75] are often due to a leaky gut.[76] As we'll discuss in the next chapter, wheat is one of the primary culprits in causing and worsening leaky gut.

Not only is there empirical evidence that removing wheat can cause autoimmune diseases to go into remission, there is also plenty of anecdotal evidence. A particularly touching story published in the *New York Times*[77] in February 2013, follows the path of a young boy with juvenile idiopathic arthritis. The standard treatments and anti-inflammatory drugs were not working for this young boy; he continued to live his life in pain, unable to run and play with his peers. Following the advice of an alternative doctor, his parents removed all gluten-containing grains from his diet. Six weeks into the plan, he experienced remission.

JOINT PAIN

Joint pain might also be impacted by wheat. The amino acid composition of grains is very similar to that of the soft tissue in your joints. When you have a leaky gut and inflammation in your body, your immune cells will rev up for the attack. In addition to attacking the grain cells, they'll also attack the soft tissue of your joints because they're so similar. This in turn leads to more inflammation. Autoimmune diseases. Pain. If you have arthritis, this is why it's particularly important for you to ditch the wheat.

"Childhood problems like learning disorders, autism, and hyperactivity can be caused by an intolerance to the proteins found in wheat."

BIG KILLERS

Internal inflammation of body tissue is associated with wheat consumption and is a precursor of a number of diseases including heart disease, cancer, diabetes, and more. [78, 79, 80, 81, 82]

WHEAT-FREE IS NOT THE CURE-ALL

We're not here to tell you that giving up wheat will be the healing elixir for all of your woes. Yes, wheat has been linked to more diseases than we have time or space to write about here. Yes, we believe everyone could benefit from a wheat-free diet. But, we also know that a nutrient-dense diet, free of other common highly-inflammatory foods, is also necessary for optimal health.

We feel confident that if you are able to clean up your diet you will see health improvements. Maybe not immediately—in fact, you probably won't see the most dramatic of results for quite some time. Yes, it warms our hearts and gives us hope when we hear of dramatic transformations the week or the month after someone has cut out wheat. But being realistic, most of us have eaten the standard American fare for far too long. Our bodies have undergone a lot of damage; it will take time to heal.

DISORDERS ASSOCIATED WITH GLUTEN INTOLERANCE:

• Abdominal Distention	• Headaches / Migraines
• Abdominal Pain	• IBS — Irritable Bowel Syndrome
• Alopecia	
• Anemia	• Impotency
• Anxiety	• Infertility
• Arthralgia or Arthropathy	• Kidney Disease
	• Liver Disease
• Arthritis	• Low Bone Mass
• Attention Deficit Disorder	• Multiple Sclerosis
• Chronic Fatigue Syndrome	• Schizophrenia and other psychiatric disorders
• Cystic Fibrosis	• Scleroderma
• Depression	• Sjogrens Syndrome
• Dermatitis	• Spontaneous Abortion and Fetal Growth Retardation
• Diabetes (Type 1)	
• Diarrhea	• Thyroid Disease
• Epilepsy	• Almost all autoimmune diseases…
• Gall Bladder Disease	

DELETE
THE WHEAT

7 REASONS WHY
YOU SHOULD

As we mentioned before, the vast majority of individuals who are sensitive to wheat do *not* exhibit any intestinal problems. (We really want that point to sink in, that's why we keep mentioning it.) However, when they cut wheat out of their diets, they experience improvement: better mood, less PMS, clearer skin, less fatigue, sharper thinking skills. Those who struggle with autoimmune diseases or mental disorders often see improvement; migraines subside, eczema and psoriasis improve, joint pain decreases, and many other improvements.

It may seem too good to be true, but I've read story after story of people who have transformed their lives and well being through a change in diet. But, it's not just stories. Oh no, we wouldn't give you just stories without science to back up these crazy claims.

THE ANTI-NUTRIENTS IN WHEAT

The problems associated with wheat all start with three "anti-nutrients": gluten, lectins, and phytates. These have been coined "anti-nutrients" because they disrupt and interfere with your body's natural ability to absorb nutrients.

After these anti-nutrients enter the body, they can cause a host of problems.

1. GLUTEN: NOT JUST A CELIAC PROBLEM

Gluten is basically the glue that holds your bread together and gives it its elastic properties. Gluten has become quite a buzz word lately because of the prevalence of "gluten-free" items now sold in stores and at restaurants throughout the world.

Celiac disease is on the rise—a 400% increase in just 50 years. For the 1% of individuals in the United States who have celiac disease, this is the protein that causes a major problem. Celiac disease is just *one* outcome of being intolerant of gluten. [83, 84, 85]

It used to be that doctors would only admit gluten was causing a problem if you had a positive biopsy showing a damaged intestinal wall. The problem with this is a biopsy is only examining a very small portion of the intestines. Damage can be done to any part of the 23 feet of small intestines you have in your body. And there currently isn't any way that we know of to test all 23 feet for damage. An intestinal biopsy is sort of a crapshoot.

We don't really know how many people suffer from non-celiac gluten sensitivity. Some doctors and researchers say they suspect *everyone* suffers from at least a small degree of gluten sensitivity. 86, 87

Why is gluten a problem for most (or all) people? Gluten is made up of two proteins: gliadin and glutenin. In everyone, gliadin causes zonulin to be released in the body. Zonulin regulates how permeable our intestinal wall is—how much liquid or gas will be able to pass through it. The more zonulin present, the more permeable your intestinal wall becomes. The more permeable your intestines are, the more partially digested food (i.e. poop) can enter in your blood stream.

It's imperative that individuals suffering from celiac disease avoid gluten. But it's also important that those who suffer from non-celiac gluten sensitivity also avoid gluten (and that means probably most everyone).

2. LECTINS: ANOTHER CAUSE FOR LEAKY GUT

Lectins are mild toxins which are found in wheat. They're basically like a plant's built-in pesticide—one of the ways a plant protects itself. Lectins aren't broken down in your gut but bind to receptors in your intestinal wall. This allows the lectins and also food particles to leech into your blood stream (again, poop in the blood).

When partially digested particles are entering your blood stream, your immune system mounts up an attack. These attacks can eventually be partially responsible for the development of autoimmune diseases, of which there are many.[88, 89]

On top of this, lectins are also implicated in causing leptin resistance. Among other things, leptin regulates your hunger cravings, and when we become resistant to leptin, this can lead to weight gain, sleep disturbances, nutritional deficiencies, and a host of other problems.[90]

Now, it's not likely that you'll completely eliminate lectins from your diet. You can go all gangbusters to get crazy healthy, but lectins are present in a *lot* of foods. You can, however, decrease your consumption of them by cutting the biggest and most detrimental offenders: those with massive quantities of lectin. Wheat is a big offender, as are all grains, legumes, and soy.[91]

One of the key take-away points in all of this is that grains are highly associated with leaky gut. When your gut isn't healthy you can't absorb nutrients so you become malnourished and more prone to disease.

3. PHYTATES: ROBBING YOU OF VITAMINS AND MINERALS

Phytates cause minerals to be "bio-unavailable." That means, when phytates are around, it makes it much more difficult for your body to utilize the vitamins and minerals that are present.[92] Phytates do this in two ways: 1) they bind up minerals and 2) they prevent minerals from being properly absorbed. They're sneaky little suckers.

Phytates are also associated with increased tooth decay—so much so that anthropologists use the level of tooth decay to determine whether a society was agricultural or a hunter/gatherer society.[93]

Now, I'm not going to tell you that phytates are all doom and gloom. There have been some studies linking them to some positive health outcomes including cancer inhibition[94] and the prevention of kidney stones.[95] But, certainly eating them in massive quantities as our typical American diet behooves of us isn't healthy.

Wheat and other grains are not the only food-stuffs that are high in phytic acid. Nuts and legumes are also quite high in phytic acid—actually they are higher in phytic acid than grains. Americans eat massive quantities of grains, nuts, legumes, and other foods that are packed with phytic acid. Not only that, but traditional preparation methods (such as soaking and sprouting) that help reduce the phytic acid content are very rarely used.

Moral of the story: some phytic acid in the diet may help to normalize cell growth and thus help inhibit cancer. But, eating huge quantities of foods with phytic acid that hasn't been prepared in such a way to break it down prior to digestion can lead to problems with malabsorption of magnesium, calcium, iron, and zinc.

(More on traditional preparation methods in chapter 7)

4. ANTI-NUTRIENTS CAUSE INFLAMMATION LEADING TO DISEASE

Inflammation is the body's natural reaction to invasion. As we explained earlier, the proteins in wheat can cause inflammation in a couple ways. First, for those with wheat allergies, the proteins themselves are interpreted by the body as invaders, and the body reacts by inflammation of the body tissue. For everyone else, the proteins in wheat are likely to cause leaky gut, putting partially digested food in the bloodstream, which is then attacked by the body the same way.

The more refined the grain, the more inflammation of your body tissue. White flour is more inflammatory than whole grain flour, but whole grain flour is still highly inflammatory.[96]

Inflammation is the predecessor to disease. When you are consistently dining on inflammatory foods, you're much more likely to succumb to degenerative diseases: asthma, cancer, arthritis, and cardiovascular disease, etc. In addition, inflammation causes your body to circulate more cholesterol to combat the inflammation. It is for this reason that inflammatory foods like sugar, wheat, and fake fats (margarine, canola oil, etc.) should be considered the dietary villains in the battle against heart disease.

Not only is eliminating wheat a good way to help cure disease, but giving up wheat and other cereal grains is a good way to help avoid disease.

5. GLUTEN ACTIVATES BRAIN RECEPTORS LEADING TO ADDICTION

Yes. True story. You might actually be having a hard time giving up wheat because you may be addicted to it. The same mechanism that causes individuals to become addicted to heroin and other opiates could also be at play when you are eating wheat.

In some people, gluten and gliad exorphins may be interacting with your opiate receptors in your brain.[97, 98] Basically, that means that your body might be treating some of the molecules in wheat the same way it would heroin.

Many scientists are pointing the finger at wheat and blaming it for binge eating disorders. When binge eaters are given the drug naloxone (a drug that is used to block heroin or morphine) they eat 30% less food.[99]

We haven't found any overtly convincing studies about this hypothesis, but going just from anecdotal evidence, it is very possible. How many times, when telling people that we don't eat any wheat, have we heard, "Oh, I could never give up wheat"? Truthfully, we had *many* false starts of giving up wheat and relapsing back with a few slices of pizza or a fresh baked muffin. I've also met many people who "tried" to give up wheat but didn't succeed.

As plausible as this theory sounds, as of now, it is just a theory. I will be very interested to see what new research is done in the coming years to address this issue.

6. GLUTEN ENTERS THE BRAIN CAUSING MENTAL DISORDERS

Mental health problems in the United States continue to increase. We're seeing more individuals with mental health problems than ever before. According to the CDC, one in five children in the United States suffer from some form of mental disorder—autism spectrum disorders, ADHD, depression, anxiety, and others.[100]

Knowing that our children are afflicted with mental disorders at these alarming rates gives us pause and makes us question whether diet is at play. You may not be surprised to hear, that many researchers are pointing their finger at wheat as, at least, one of the contributing factors to this increase in mental disorders.

After gluten has been broken down, it can cross the blood-brain barrier: wheat can cause the immune system to attack the nervous system. This explains why gluten is thought to be a contributor to mental disorders.

Researchers began to notice the gluten-schizophrenia correlation quite some time ago. During World War II, researchers noted that as gluten rations decreased, so did prevalence of hospital admissions for schizophrenia (seen across countries).[101]

Then, in the 50's, researchers noticed there was a much greater prevalence of schizophrenic and psychotic individuals among their celiac patients. Furthermore, when wheat was eliminated from the diet of schizophrenic patients, a marked improvement was often seen. When wheat was re-added to the patient's diet, they deteriorated once again.[102]

The research has continued to pile up with recent studies linking wheat consumption to schizophrenia.[103, 104, 105, 106]

Autism spectrum disorders and children with ADD often see improvement when eliminating wheat as well.[107, 108]

Now, we doubt gluten is the sole reason for schizophrenia and other mental disorders. Obviously, not everyone who eats wheat ends up with schizophrenia. But it is likely that it is one of the variables that has contributed to the rise in mental disorders in recent years.[109, 110, 111]

7. WHEAT TURNS INTO SUGAR WHICH LEADS TO WEIGHT PROBLEMS

When it comes to the connection between wheat and weight gain, there are a number of different things at play. One of the big ones is the insulin spike that grains cause. When you eat wheat, it is broken down to sugar in your body. This causes the pancreas to secrete insulin. After the insulin spike comes the blood sugar "crash." When your levels crash, you're left feeling hungry. So, you eat more, probably a carbohydrate rich snack to fill the void. This causes you to eat more over the course of the day than if you were consuming foods that kept your insulin levels stable.

Another problem with this cycle is that when insulin levels are continually high (as they often are in a Western diet), you *store fat* instead of burning fat. Two slices of whole wheat (or whole grain) bread will raise your blood sugar more than a SNICKERS® bar. One slice of white bread or one bagel will also raise your blood sugar levels more than a SNICKERS®

bar.[112] Don't be fooled; just because it's labeled "whole grain" does not mean it's healthy.

Of course, wheat is not the only problem with weight gain. Other grains and sugar—along with messed-up hormones from a lifetime of poor eating habits—are big factors in weight gain as well.

"Two slices of whole wheat (or whole grain) bread will raise your blood sugar more than a SNICKERS®"

I was so excited and happy to have clear skin.

I have had horrible acne on my face for years and have tried everything in the traditional medicine world to treat it. I then started going to a Naturopath and started natural ways to get my body healthy... After the three week cleanse my acne was pretty much nonexistent, I was so excited and happy to have clear skin.

The first food I reintroduced was bread and my acne returned. I also felt awful; I was nauseous, tired and cranky. So I decided to take wheat back out of my diet again for three weeks then reintroduce and I had the same results.

I know the day after when I have had something with wheat or gluten because my face breaks out. Even though I am very careful not to eat anything with it in it, it can be hard sometimes. I have so much more energy now and I am actually starting to lose weight when I hadn't lost more than 5 pounds in three years.

—Megan

WHEAT'S THE PROBLEM?

HOW TO TEST FOR PROBLEMS WITH WHEAT

Perhaps if you are like me (Trisha), despite your love of wheat products, you suspect (or are convinced) your body has a problem with wheat. Or perhaps if you are like both of us, after reading the research on all the potential problems that are linked to wheat, you believe it is best to stay away from wheat anyway.

Either way, having your doctor run tests to determine wheat sensitivity can be helpful. It's nice to be able to waive an "official" test showing you're intolerant to wheat in front of the wheat-loving nay-sayers who would otherwise deter you from a new lifestyle.

Having test results can also be a helpful motivator in the future when you have that urge to pick up the phone and order a late-night pizza.

TESTS TO DETERMINE WHEAT SENSITIVITY

Are there ways to definitively determine whether you have a problem with wheat? Yes and no. Testing is available, but it isn't comprehensive. It's complicated, as are most things in life (truth!). Below are some of the tests that you can ask for if you suspect you have a problem with gluten sensitivity.

1. A STANDARD ALLERGY SCRATCH OR INTRADERMAL TEST

These tests can give you some insight, though often people who have problems with wheat don't react to this test. Surprisingly, this is one test I (Trisha) did react to.

Prior to this test, I had been mostly gluten-free, but I splurged from time to time. Since taking this test, I don't knowingly consume wheat. I've found since I've given up wheat, when I do consume it, my body lets me know it does not like it. It is normal, after giving up wheat for a length of time, for your body to become more sensitive to it—it means your body has begun the healing process.

2. ANTIBODY BLOOD TESTS (SPECIFICALLY IGG AND IGA)

These test look for immune system reactions. It may or may not mean you have a problem with wheat, but it would be a clue if your levels were elevated. I (Trisha) also had this test done, but my levels were not elevated.

3. THE HLA-DQ TEST

This is a genetic test, and it's much more sensitive. It picks up problems in many more people than the antibody tests. If you carry at least one of a certain kind of gene you are at a fairly high risk of having or developing celiac disease. (There are likely other genes that are at play that determine whether a person will develop celiac disease.)

4. AN INTESTINAL BIOPSY

This used to be the considered the gold standard for testing for celiac disease, but it's not a very good test as it isn't very accurate. Your intestines cover a *huge* surface area. When doctors do this biopsy, they are looking for damage to the villi in your intestines. A biopsy is a test of a minuscule portion of your intestines. The problem is, there are a *lot* of false negatives. Some people have many intestinal biopsies done over the course of their life before one comes back positive. Think of all of the damage that gluten has done to that person's body in that time frame because some doctors insist that there must be a positive biopsy before a diagnosis can be made.

5. THERE ARE NEW SALIVA AND BLOOD TESTS FROM CRYEX LABORATORIES[113]

These tests for detecting gluten sensitivities are quite promising. From initial reports, these tests are much better at detecting problems with gluten, but only time will tell if they can truly do the job. The biggest problem with Cryex tests is it's doubtful that your insurance will cover them, and again, there can be false negatives.

THE BEST TEST FOR GLUTEN SENSITIVITIES

What's the best way to tell if you have a problem with wheat? Give it up. Give wheat up for a minimum of 2 months with strict adherence. Some people can tell a difference within days, but it can take months for gluten and other wheat toxins to clear out of your system. Months. Sometimes longer than 2 months.

Even if you don't experience alleviation in your problems, if you have diseases like an autoimmune disease, infertility, or other diseases that demonstrate long-term damage, we'd strongly urge you to cut out all wheat indefinitely.

A last note, if you are planning to have testing done, be sure to get your testing done prior to giving up wheat. The tests will be more reliable if the proteins from wheat are currently in your system. If you give up gluten-containing grains and then decide to add them back for testing, you may experience some, umm… unpleasantness.

"Having test results can also be a helpful motivator in the future when you have that urge to pick up the phone and order a late-night pizza."

FAQ

FREQUENTLY ASKED QUESTIONS ABOUT WHEAT

Isn't the problem with wheat just because it is so processed? What if I grind my own wheat?

No doubt, the highly processed wheat that is in our foods today is a problem, but the problem is not just the fact that it's processed. Please refer to Chapter 5 to read more about the problems associated with wheat. All of the problematic proteins are still present in whole grain wheat and have the potential to cause the same problems. But if you're grinding your own wheat, it's certainly healthier than eating Twinkies® and Ding-Dong's.®

What about traditionally prepared wheat? Doesn't that solve potential problems?

We've heard this question numerous times. Someone will claim, "I heard that you can still eat sourdough bread if you have celiac disease or are gluten intolerant." So, here's our spiel on traditional preparation of grains.

If you choose to eat grains, we'd definitely suggest preparing them traditionally as they will help you digest them more easily. Traditional preparation does not mean picking up a loaf of (fake) sourdough bread from the store. It means taking the time to actually start a wild yeast starter, soaking, or sprouting your grains. There are some great resources online to get you started in this process. This is much healthier than eating commercially available grains.

To date, we've found three studies that have examined celiac patients' tolerance of sourdough bread.[114, 115, 116]

- The first thing to note about these studies is that they used a very small sample size—just 5, 8, and 17 subjects in each of the studies. This is hardly enough to base global recommendations upon for everyone suffering from gluten intolerance or celiac disease.

- The type of sourdough used in these lab studies would be impossible to replicate in your own home. This bread was created in a lab under very specific conditions, with very specific procedures, and it underwent much testing prior to consumption.

- There have been no long-term studies to determine long lasting implications. These studies only looked at immediate acute intestinal response.

- Our biggest concern about these studies is what they *don't* prove. We'd argue there is much more at risk than simply gastrointestinal distress when eating wheat and other grains. Our previous chapters outline these potential problems.

In the making of sourdough bread, *some* of the problematic proteins and enzymes in wheat (phytate, lectins, and gluten) are deactivated, and this is certainly a good thing.

Here's the rundown on how traditionally preparing grains impacts the phytates, lectins, gluten, and enzyme inhibitors. *Some* of the phytates may be deactivated in sourdough bread, but the majority of it remains intact. Enzyme inhibitors in wheat are mostly deactivated when traditionally preparing grains which allows you to digest the grains much more easily. Traditional preparation can also deactivate some of the lectins, but some also remain. Likewise, some or much of the gluten can be deactivated, but it's likely that there is at least some that remains (unless, of course, you're making laboratory bread that's gone through extensive testing).

Won't I be missing out on a lot of vitamins and minerals if I give up wheat?

You won't be missing out on any vitamins and minerals at all as long as you replace your wheat consumption with real, whole, healthy foods. Not only is wheat *not* the best source of vitamins, the anti-nutrients in wheat and other grains *stop* your body from absorbing the vitamins that are found in these foods.

People often worry about not getting enough B vitamins, including B6, folate, and thiamin. These B vitamins are actually available in the same or higher amounts in many other foods. For example, Vitamin B6 is found in higher concentrations in salmon, chicken breast, avocado, spinach, and tuna, just to name a few food sources.

Folate is more abundant in asparagus, avocado, spinach, Brussels sprouts, Romaine lettuce, and more.

Thiamin is found in greater amounts in tuna, sunflower seeds, black beans, many herbs, spices, and other sources.

Beyond this, it's actually possible—in fact, quite probable—that your body will be able to absorb the nutrients you are ingesting from other foods more readily when you eliminate wheat from your diet. It makes much more sense to get your nutrients from fruits, vegetables, real healthy fats, and pastured meats than it does to depend on nutrient-poor, vitamin-leaching wheat!

With all this talk about how wheat has changed, I'm wondering: Was ancient wheat good for us?

That's a good question. It depends on what you compare it to. Here are our thoughts, given the research we've read.

Consuming a moderate amount of ancient wheat, using traditional preparation methods, in a person that isn't suffering from different problems (like autoimmune diseases, heart disease, high blood pressure, cancer, etc.) probably wouldn't be too bad. Unfortunately, today there are so many of us who have eaten the standard American diet for so long that we've likely damaged our bodies to the point that complete abstinence from wheat, even ancient wheat varieties, is beneficial.

Is traditionally prepared ancient wheat "good" for us when compared to Twinkies (duh)? Or even compared to a slice of whole wheat bread from the store? Yes. But, is ancient wheat as good for us as grass-fed beef, fresh vegetables, and butter from grass-fed cows? Nope—it's not nearly as good of a source of nutrition.

Also, finding an ancient source of wheat that's totally unblemished from the current practices of transgenic breeding may be difficult. Even those selling ancient wheat can't guarantee that there hasn't been cross-contamination with modern wheat. For us, finding the wheat, grinding the wheat, and preparing it myself sounds a bit tedious even if we wanted to try it.

TESTIMONIAL

"the brain fog which I'd been experiencing for nearly two years began to clear up."

I cut out gluten earlier this year as part of my potential healing protocol for apparent thyroid and adrenal issues. First I switched from standard wheat to spelt bread and cut down on other wheat in my diet. A few months later I cut out all wheat and the brain fog which I'd been experiencing for nearly two years began to clear up. I had a few times of eating wheat after that, and the grogginess and foggy head returned just as fast. That was enough evidence to continue being gluten-free. Since then I have had some accidental moments of getting some in my system, but that has been rare and I notice an overall improvement in my health this year.

—Soli from iBelieveInButter.wordpress.com

IS EATING WHEAT-FREE BIBLICAL?

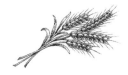

RECONCILING A WHEAT-FREE DIET WITH A BREAD-FILLED FAITH

WHEAT AND BREAD IN THE BIBLE

WHEN FAITH AND FOOD COLLIDE

For most people, the question of whether wheat-free eating is "Biblical" has never entered their minds. But for others, this is the question where their faith and their health collide. It certainly was for us.

As followers of Jesus Christ, the Bible is indispensable to us. Jesus taught His followers that the Scriptures can never be broken (John 10:35)—the truths expressed in the Bible will endure until the end of the world (Matthew 5:18). The Old Testament was the basis of Christ's teachings (Matt. 7:12; Mark 12:29-31; Luke 16:31), and He promised the Holy Spirit would inspire the New Testament (John 14:26, 15:26-27, 16:12-15).

It follows for all Christians: if the Scriptures were of central importance to the Redeemer, they are important for those He redeemed.

With this in mind, what does the Bible have to say about wheat and bread?

WHEAT: A STAPLE OF LIFE

The Bible was written in an agrarian culture where wheat and bread were commonplace.

Wheat was a part of the regular commerce of ancient Israel (1 Kings 5:11; 2 Chr. 2:10; Amos 8:5-6), and bread was part of ordinary meals (Gen. 14:18, 25:34, 27:17, 37:25, 43:31; Ex. 16:3, 18:12). Harvesting and threshing wheat was an annual event for the people of Israel (Gen. 30:14; Ex. 34:22; Judges 6:11, 15:1; Ruth 1:22, 2:23; 1 Sam. 6:13, 12:17; 1 Chr. 21:20). In fact, the Feast of Weeks (also called Pentecost) was an annual festival that coincided with the wheat harvest. As such, every year, faithful Hebrew men would come to Jerusalem to praise God for His faithfulness, bringing in another harvest of wheat.

In the Scriptures, a good wheat harvest and abundant bread was a sign of God's blessing (Ex. 23:25; Ps. 81:16, 147:14; Joel 2:24). A poor wheat harvest was a sign of God's curse (Jer. 12:13; Lam. 4:4; Joel 1:11).

During Israel's 40 years in the desolate wilderness, they did not eat ordinary bread (Deut. 29:6), but instead ate manna from heaven, which was called the "bread of angels" (Ex. 16:4, 15,

32; Ps. 78:25, 105:40). This changed, however, once Israel arrived in Canaan. Israel anticipated the land of Canaan would be a land abundant in wheat and barley (Deut. 8:8), and it most certainly was.

WHEAT: REGULARLY USED IN WORSHIP

Wheat and bread were part of the religious life of Israel. A special bread called showbread was placed in the tabernacle at all times (Ex. 25:30, 35:13). Sheaves of wheat and baked bread were acceptable sacrifices to God (Ex. 29:2; Lev. 7:13; Num. 5:15; 1 Chr. 21:23; Ezek. 45:14). Passover specifically was a time when Israel was commanded to eat unleavened bread (Ex. 12:8). Directly following Passover was the Feast of Unleavened Bread, celebrated for seven days (Ex. 13:6, 23:15, 34:18; Lev. 23:6; Deut. 16:3; Ezek. 45:21).

WHEAT IN THE LIFE OF JESUS

Jesus also ate bread during His life. On two occasions, Jesus miraculously multiplied a few loaves of bread into enough food to feed thousands (Matt. 14:19, 15:36; Mark 6:41, 8:6; Luke 9:16; John 6:11). He taught His disciples to pray, "Give us this day our daily bread" (Matt. 6:11; Luke 11:3). He ate bread with His disciples even after His resurrection (Luke 24:30; John 21:9). He used bread during the Last Supper to speak of His body (Matt. 26:26; Mark 14:22; Luke 22:19). He referred to Himself as the "true bread" from Heaven and "the bread of life" (John 6:32, 48).

WHEAT: NOT ALWAYS ASSOCIATED WITH ABUNDANCE

While wheat was a staple of life and a provision from God in ancient Israel, it was not necessarily associated with a time of plenty. In times of great scarcity, wheat and other grains were often the only crops available (Gen. 41:53-57; 1 Kings 17:8-16). It was only in times of severe famine that even the bread would run out (Amos 4:6; Joel 1:17).

When the prophet Ezekiel was commanded to "act out" a prophetic sign about Israel and Judah's exile, he was told to lay on his side for 430 days—that's a year and a couple months— and told to eat nothing but bread cooked over cow dung (Ezekiel 4). To all the exiles watching Ezekiel in bewilderment, God was sending a message about the coming siege against Jerusalem: "Son of man, I will make food very scarce in Jerusalem… Lacking food and water, people will look at one another in terror, and they will waste away under their punishment" (Ez. 4:16-17). In Ezekiel's demonstration, eating nothing but wheat bread was a symbol of a meager, malnourished diet.

(It is ironic that stores today sell "Ezekiel Bread" as if it is God's holy recipe for great bread. In the text of Ezekiel, it was a symbol of famine and punishment, not plenty. But if you do eat Ezekiel bread, go varsity and toast it over flaming poop. You'll have our deepest admiration.)

My point is not that Ezekiel's bread was itself a curse—after all, it kept him alive for over a year—but that it was a symbol of judgment and great scarcity.

In contrast, an abundance of meat and wine were indicators of great plenty. Feasts and festivals were often accompanied with the eating of meat (Luke 15:23). After leaving Egypt and entering the vast wilderness, Israel longed for the pots of meat in Egypt (Ex.16:3).

IN SUMMARY

Bread was very important to the daily life of God's people. It was an assumed staple of life. But while bread was a provision from God, it was not necessarily always a symbol of richness or abundance. Bread alone was a meager meal.

With these facts in mind, can a Christian who takes the Bible seriously walk away from wheat and still honor the traditions of God's people?

WHEAT IS A PROVISION, NOT AN OBLIGATION

DOES GOD LOVE GLUTEN?

Is a wheat-free diet "Biblical?" At first glance it would seem it isn't.

Let's be clear what we mean by "Biblical." For the purposes of this chapter, we are not asking whether the Bible *endorses* a wheat-free diet. It clearly does not. Wheat is everywhere in the Bible. Rather, the question is: Does the Bible *obligate* us to eat wheat, to treat wheat like a staple of life?

Or putting it another way: Are those eating a wheat-free diet somehow out-of-step with the way God wants us to eat?

USING WINE AS AN ANALOGY

In the Christian world, there is no shortage of disagreement about whether a Christian is allowed to drink alcohol. I (Luke), for one, enjoy drinking wine, but many of my fellow Christians would find my enjoyment of alcohol questionable at best.

Bible-believing Christians do agree that drunkenness is sinful (Deut. 21:20; Hosea 4:10-11; Amos 6:4-7; Prov. 20:1, 23:29-35; 1 Pet. 4:1-5; Eph. 5:18), and there are plenty of circumstances where altogether abstaining from alcohol is wise (Prov. 31:4; Rom. 14:15, 21).

However, one cannot read the Bible and escape the conclusion that God counts wine and other alcoholic drinks as blessings.[117]

God blessed Israel with wine for obedient and wise living (Deut. 7:13, 11:14; Prov. 3:9-10), and the loss of wine was evidence of God's curse (Deut. 28:39; Hosea 9:2; Joel 1:10; Amos 5:11; Mic. 6:15; Zeph. 1:13; Hag. 1:11). God even tells His people that abundant wine is one of the blessings of the age to come. On the day God wipes away every tear, He "will make for all peoples a feast of rich food, a feast of well-aged wine, of rich food full of marrow, or aged wine well refined" (Is. 24:6; cf. Amos 9:14; Jer. 31:12; Joel 2:24-25).

Like wheat and bread, wine was an acceptable sacrifice to give to God in the form of drink offerings (Ex. 29:40; Lev. 23:13; Num. 15:5; Deut. 18:4; Ezra 6:9). The Levites received wine for themselves from the tithes given by worshipers (Num. 18:30).

Wine was a drink of celebration. God gives wine to "gladden the heart of man" (Ps. 104:14). God even *invited* His people to celebrate in His presence by drinking wine. Year after year, those who traveled a great distance to Jerusalem were told to use their tithe money to buy "whatever you desire—oxen or sheep or wine or strong drink, whatever your appetite craves. And you shall eat there before the Lord your God and rejoice, you and your household" (Deut. 14:26).

Paul counsels his disciple Timothy, "No longer drink only water, but use a little wine for the sake of your stomach and your frequent ailments" (1 Timothy 5:23). This home-remedy for poor digestion has actually been confirmed by modern studies. Fermented drinks like beer, sherry, or wine are powerful stimulants for gastric acid secretion[118, 119] and can even speed up the emptying of the stomach.[120] Red wine also contains polyphenols that trigger the release of nitric oxide which relaxes the stomach wall, thus optimizing digestion.[121]

Jesus Himself banqueted with wine to demonstrate the joy of the nearness of the kingdom of God. For His first miracle, Jesus miraculously produced more than one hundred and twenty gallons of fine wine for a wedding feast (John 2:6-11). One of the marks of Jesus' ministry was His table fellowship with notorious sinners and eager learners (Luke 5:29, 7:48, 10:39, 11:37-52, 14:4, 15:2, 19:1-9, 10:39). And yes, these feasts often included the drinking of wine.

"John the Baptist has come eating no bread and drinking no wine," Jesus told the crowds, but "the Son of Man has come eating and drinking" (Luke 7:33-34). In contrast to John the Baptist, a man of the wilderness who often fasted (Matt. 9:14; Mark 1:6), Jesus was known for His joyful feasting—so much so His critics unjustly called Him "a glutton and a drunkard" (Luke 7:34). Through the presence of Jesus, the kingdom of heaven was at hand; it was a time of celebration.

"Obligation does not follow from blessing"

Last, Jesus chose wine to represent His blood. During Jesus' last Passover meal, several cups of wine were shared among the disciples (Luke 22:17-18, 20). Right after the meal, Jesus picked up a cup of wine, gave a word of thanks to His Father, and then said, "Drink of it, all of you, for this is my blood of the covenant, which is poured out for many for the forgiveness of sins. I tell you I will not drink again of this fruit of the vine until that day when I drink it new with you in my Father's kingdom" (Matt. 26:27-29).

THE MAIN POINT: ATTITUDE IS EVERYTHING

If we take our cues from the Scriptures, our attitude about wine should be that it is a *blessing* from God. As much as wine can be abused (and it is), it is a blessing nonetheless, and our attitude ought to reflect that. As Christians who take the Scriptures seriously, we should be able to praise God for this good gift.

But note: just because wine is a blessing does not mean we *must* drink it. No Bible-believing Christian would claim, "The Bible says wine is a blessing, so *not drinking* is sinful." No. *Obligation does not follow from blessing.*

Many things in the Bible are labeled as blessings. Marriage and children are blessings, but this does not *obligate* all to be married or have children. Wealth is a blessing, but this does not *obligate* all to be rich. *Obligation does not follow from blessing.*

The same can be said of wheat and bread. Yes, the Bible speaks of wheat and bread as blessings from God. But this speaks to our *attitude*, not our obligations.

Putting it another way, we can wholeheartedly affirm that God calls wheat a blessing, but if we conclude from this that those who don't eat wheat are *failing* to live up to God's standard, we have taken things too far. To make all blessings obligations misreads the Bible.

THE HEART OF THE MATTER

Christians are right to want the conclusions of modern medicine to bow to the authority of Scripture. If the undeniable conclusions of Scripture clash with the theories of modern science, it is *science* that must reexamine its facts, not the Bible.

When you look at the negative health impact of wheat—potentially even ancient varieties of wheat—many Christians scratch their heads and ask, "Are you saying that wheat is a *curse* when the Bible calls it a *blessing*?" Some Christians, when confronted with the negative health impact of wheat, will say, "The Bible calls wheat a blessing. God commanded His people to eat it on a variety of occasions. God commanded His people to grow it and give it to Him as an offering. If you are saying wheat is a curse, you are denying what the Bible overwhelmingly says about it."

We wholeheartedly agree. The Bible certainly speaks of wheat in a generally positive light. To deny this is to ignore or deny what Scripture says about it. Wheat is most certainly *not* a "curse."

However, it is important to define our terms. Just as we should not ignore or deny Scripture in favor of science, neither should we try to fit Scripture into science's mold. The Bible was not written in modern scientific language. When Scripture says wheat is a blessing, unless we have biblical reason to do so, we should not interpret "blessing" to mean "without imperfection" or "something that the body cannot live without" or "nutritionally superior," or even "nutritionally excellent."

To clarify, there are many reasons why the Bible might label wheat a blessing that have *nothing* to do with nutrition. Bread can fill a man's stomach, satisfying his hunger and give him energy (Psalm 104:15). Wheat is a robust crop, widely available and able to be grown in a variety of climates. Products made from wheat are also satisfying in taste and texture. Any or all of these factors could make wheat a blessing, but we should not feel the need to interpret the Bible through the language of modern nutrition.

Where does this leave us when it comes to God and nutrition? The fact remains that God not only planted His people in a place abundant with wheat but also commanded them, at times, to consume it. The fact also remains that God knew there was gluten and other potentially harmful proteins in wheat. Even if we believe ancient wheat was nutritionally superior to modern wheat (and it was), we must still face the fact that God knowingly provided His people with gluten-filled grains.

We draw a number of conclusions from this. First and foremost, if a Christian eschews all wheat for health reasons, they must not carry the attitude that they are somehow smarter than God or that God "got this one wrong." We should never call a curse what God calls a blessing. When a Christian sees "amber waves of grain" (minus any thoughts about unwise modern mutations), they should say in their heart, "Praise God for providing for us."

Second, we should be reminded not to idolize nutrition. If God can knowingly feed His people food with potentially unhelpful qualities and still call it a blessing, we should not be too quick to make ideal nutrition the be-all and end-all of our lives. God certainly didn't. The kingdom of God is not ultimately about what we eat or drink, but about righteousness, peace, and joy in the Holy Spirit (Romans 14:17).

Third, it is possible to call something a blessing knowing that there are aspects of it that are not beneficial. Wine is a blessing, but too much of it will cause drunkenness and multiple health problems. Orange roughy and yellowfin tuna are tasty kosher fish, but too much of them will raise mercury levels in your body. And yes, wheat is a blessing in many respects, but this does not mean that it cannot do damage to your body. God is satisfied calling these things blessings despite the potential negative impacts, and so should we.

Last, if we give up wheat because modern diets have wreaked havoc on our bodies, we should never lose touch with the agrarian world in which the Bible was written—a world where God brought His people into a "good land...of wheat and barley" (Deuteronomy 8:8), a world where God promised to fill His people with "the finest of the wheat" (Psalm 81:16; 147:14), a world where Jesus called Himself "the Bread of Life" (John 6:48).

TESTIMONIAL

"My psoriasis has stayed away and my arthritis seems to be gone for good as well."

I started eating wheat free nearly 2 years ago after several members in my family had tried it with fantastic health results. I decided to give it a try. I stuck with it, with a few slip-up's every now and then. But, when I finally stuck to it without any cheats I began to see results. About 8 weeks into my gluten-free diet my arthritis symptoms began to subside and I noticed I needed fewer medications. The next thing I noticed was that my psoriasis had vanished. I eat a clean diet with no wheat. My psoriasis has stayed away and my arthritis seems to be gone for good as well.

—CJL

DOES GOD HAVE A DIET PLAN?

HEALTH AND
THE KOSHER DIET

A trend among some Christians today is the desire to eat what they believe to be the "Biblical diet."

In the Old Testament, God called some foods "clean" and other foods "unclean." Many foods were forbidden: pigs, dogs, donkeys, camels, bats, bears, lobsters, hawks, lizards, frogs, and many other animals. Some Christians today still follow these dietary practices: some from the conviction that God still *demands* it, others from the conviction that kosher eating is simply *healthy*—the "ideal diet" given by the Maker Himself.

Some Christians take this a step further: not only did God forbid certain foods because they are unhealthy, but God also planted Israel in a region of the world that produced an abundance of ideal foods. The staple crops and livestock of ancient Israel were not only "clean," but they are the *best* foods for sustaining human life. These Christians hold to the belief that a Mediterranean kosher diet, similar to that of the ancient Hebrews, is the best and wisest diet available to us.

Space does not permit us to tackle the question here about whether unclean foods are still forbidden for the follower of Christ. Rather, the point of this chapter is to address the health assumption. Has God prescribed a specific diet for health reasons?

CORRECTING AN ASSUMPTION

Those who follow a kosher diet for health reasons generally believe one of two things:

1. Some believe a kosher diet was the optimal diet then and remains the optimal diet now.

2. Others believe the kosher diet was optimal then, but since we've invented better preservation and preparation methods, the ideal diet today is broader than it was back then.

However, health is only an *assumption* people bring to the text of the Bible. *Nowhere* in the Bible does God state that physical health is the reason for a kosher diet. *Nowhere.* God did not say that crabs are unclean because they are bottom-feeders. So are carp and halibut, but they are not forbidden. Why is the honeybee unclean but honeybee vomit (a.k.a. honey) is not? We are simply not told.

The reasons for the distinctions between clean and unclean animals are unknown to us, but a careful study of ancient cultures might give us some clues. For instance, in Exodus 23:19, God forbids the boiling of a young goat in the milk of its mother. No reason for this prohibition is given, but we know from extra-Biblical sources that this was a type of animal sacrifice done during the worship of idols. It is possible God forbids this because of its association with pagan practices. One popular theory says unclean animals were forbidden because they were totems of the primitive clans of Israel: the clean-unclean distinction was God's way of separating Israel from its idolatrous past.[122]

"*Nowhere in the Bible does God state that physical health is the reason for a kosher diet. Nowhere.*"

How does this bear on the discussion about wheat? We cannot assume that God placed His people in a region ideal for growing wheat because he believed wheat was somehow an ideal crop. There are more than 130 species of plants that grow in Israel, all of which are technically kosher, but are nonetheless toxic, even deadly.[123] Just because it was kosher and available to eat in Israel did not mean it was also healthy.

THERE IS NO BIBLICALLY NUTRITIONAL DIET

Most Christians do not follow a kosher diet. But even if one holds to the belief that God still forbids certain foods, it does *not* follow that God forbids these foods for health reasons. Additionally, just because other foods are not "unclean" does not mean that all allowed foods are thereby healthy. Optimal physical health is simply not part of the Biblical discussion. Nowhere does God prescribe a diet as the ideal healthy diet.

THE BREAD
OF LIFE

WHEAT-FREE COMMUNION?

Undoubtedly, the question of taking Communion (what some call the Eucharist) is of great concern for those who do not eat wheat. Taking the Lord's Supper is one of the most common and celebrated sacraments of the church. Christ Himself told His disciples to break bread in remembrance of Him (1 Cor. 11:24). If there ever was an endorsement of bread in the Bible, this would be it.

The Lord's Supper has sadly been a point of contention and disagreement over the centuries. For instance: Should the bread be leavened or unleavened? This was one of the great theological differences between the Eastern Orthodox and the Roman Catholic churches and one of the contributing factors of the Great Schism of AD 1054. Another example: How is Christ present in the Supper? Is the bread transfigured into the body of Christ? Is He present in some spiritual fashion? Is He only memorialized? This was a major point of disagreement between

Protestant and Catholic during the Reformation, and even among Protestants.

With the rise of health concerns about wheat, churches have had to face another question of practice: Should Communion bread be made of wheat or can it be made of other substances?

Many churches leave this matter up to pastoral judgment. Many congregants in the Missouri Synod of the Lutheran Church, for instance, are allowed to take gluten-free bread as long as the bread has been consecrated by the pastor. Other denominations, from Presbyterian to Methodist to Baptist to Anglican, are also beginning to offer gluten-free options for Communion.

Canon law of the Catholic Church states that Communion hosts *must* be made from wheat, not any other grain. But even for churches that require wheat bread, there are many "gluten-free hosts" that have been manufactured—still made from wheat but with less than 20 gluten parts per million (compliant with FDA gluten-free guidelines).

There are many interesting theological questions churches should ask when it comes to Communion bread. Some argue the bread should be unleavened to keep with the Biblical picture of being an "unleavened (pure) people" (1 Cor. 5:7-8). Some argue the original bread of the Last Supper was made from barley. Others say it was made of wheat grain. Some say we should use wheat bread in Communion to be in keeping with the Biblical picture of Christ as a grain of wheat: sown, buried, and rising to new life (John 12:24).

While all of these questions are worth considering, for our family, three truths guided our understanding in this more than anything else.

1. While different arguments could be made about the exact kind of bread eaten at the Last Supper, the Bible is silent about it. No point is made to specify the exact kind of bread eaten by the disciples on the night before Jesus' crucifixion. If the Bible is not going to specify the exact kind of bread used, it is best not to be dogmatic about what kind of bread we use.

   If the goal is to eat the same sort of bread consumed by the disciples at the Last Supper, perhaps we should ask if all grain for Communion bread should be grown in Israel. Should we require the bread be made by hand? Should we require the bread be made from ancient einkorn or emmer wheat? Taken to an extreme, desiring to "eat the bread Jesus ate" becomes pretty ridiculous pretty fast.

2. The beauty of using both bread and wine for the Lord's Supper is that Jesus chose elements that would have been common table food and drink all throughout the Roman world. In doing this, Jesus created a very accessible sacrament: all in the church can eat at the Lord's Table.

One of the points of using such accessible elements was to draw people near, not alienate. In fact, when wealthier people in the church later used the Lord's Supper as an opportunity to feast and get drunk to the exclusion of those who had no food, God severely disciplined them. Paul said when we eat the Lord's Supper and we don't acknowledge the Lord's body, the church, we are eating and drinking in an "unworthy manner" (1 Cor. 11:27).

By extension, to alienate those in the body of Christ who have severe gluten sensitivities because of an insistence on using wheat full of gluten breaks the spirit of the Supper.

3. Whatever personal convictions we might have about the kind of bread that is eaten, submission to the local church is important in this matter. It is not up for individual Christians to decide how they want to treat the Lord's Supper—it is, after all, *His* table, not ours.

This is why it is important for Christians to submit to local church leadership when it comes to this issue. Efforts should be made for church leaders to be made aware of the potential health concerns—for both celiacs and others—so that decisions can be reached as a community.

TESTIMONIAL

"Going gluten-free has been the most positive change my family has made..."

Prior to changing my diet and eliminating wheat and gluten completely, I was extremely sick. I went from doctor to doctor, and not once did a traditional doctor, using Western Medicine, suggest making a dietary change. I was simply prescribed new pills and subjected to invasive test after test.

After getting progressively worse and becoming completely bedridden for nearly a year, and in and out of the hospital regularly, I was ready to give up. My husband convinced me to give one more doctor a try, and I agreed. We went to see a Naturopathic Doctor and one of the first things that he did was make a suggestion to address my diet and stop consuming all gluten products. I wasn't convinced that simply giving up gluten would work to help me. After all, if it was as easy as changing my diet, wouldn't one of the *countless doctors or specialists I'd seen in the past have suggested this? But I was shocked, and still am at times today, that I began to get better.*

In just a short few weeks, I was able to get out of bed and spend time with my family, hang out with my children, and even take a short walk. Seeing more progress by making this one simple change than I'd seen in years of therapy with pills, procedures, and even surgeries, finally gave me the motivation that I needed to continue. Over the course of about 6-8 weeks, I saw even bigger changes—my skin issues that required Rx steroid creams to control went away. My gastroparesis/delayed gastric emptying got better and my frequent, daily bouts of severe nausea and vomiting started to dissipate. Even things like my attitude and general happiness changed for the positive; I wasn't as "down." And my weight stabilized too—no more fighting the scale or crazy weight loss diets. I finally hit a healthy, natural weight that has maintained itself without diet or hunger (I eat ALL the time!). And my blood work even stopped showing countless deficiencies as it had prior; my Naturopath explained this was due to the wheat no longer stopping my body from absorbing the nutrients it needed.

Once my health began showing signs of improvement, we made a change for the entire family, and while not everyone was as obviously sick before cutting out wheat completely, we saw changes in everyone. My children behaved better, and my school age son finally quiet having nighttime accidents within a month of making the change. Another son's constant stomach ache complaints went away as did regular and severe gas pains. Even my husband makes claims of general overall better health and mental moods.

In the end, the best part about going gluten free for me was knowing I was not crazy! After years and years of frequent emergency room visits and doctor's trips, I'd began to think I was absolutely nuts. No one could pinpoint a reason that I had gotten so sick and ended up bedridden the way that I was. Physicians, as well as family members, slowly gave up supporting my battle to get well, making assumptions that I was just making things up. I now realize how important it is to consume the right foods for my body, and wheat (or anything containing gluten) is not one of those "right foods." I wish that someone would have sat me down years ago and suggested giving up gluten for better health. Going gluten-free has been the most positive change my family has made for better physical and emotional health. Instead of continuing to cover up my gluten-based medical issues, my body has finally been given a real chance at healing itself.

—Krystyna Thomas from SpringMountainLiving.com

IN CONCLUSION

WHAT DOES WHEAT-FREE LIVING HAVE TO DO WITH OUR FAITH?

Ultimately, as Christians, we stand on the truth that the kingdom of God is not about what we eat or drink (Rom. 14:17). Neither *eating* wheat nor *avoiding* it is a barometer of spirituality. "Man does not live by bread alone, but man lives by every word that comes from the mouth of the Lord." (Deut. 8:3).

TO SUMMARIZE

- The Bible speaks of bread and wheat as provisions from God. Wheat was a staple crop for ancient Israel. Our attitudes should reflect this: God gave us wheat as one of many means to sustain life.

- In the Bible, wheat was not always associated with abundance and prosperity, but was often a fallback crop that would sustain God's people when nothing else would. For this, we should be thankful but also be attentive to the fact that wheat is far from being presented as an "ideal" food.

- Though bread and wheat were blessings, *obligation* does not follow from blessing. Many things are labeled blessings, but this does not obligate us to consume them, own them, or use them. If Christians are not looked down on for not drinking wine, neither are they required by God to eat wheat.

- Nowhere in the Bible are we taught that God has prescribed an ideal diet. The Scriptures give no recipe for ideal nutrition. Even in the making of Communion bread, wheat nor any other specific grain is prescribed by the Scriptures.

CHRISTIANS AND WHEAT-FREE LIVING

When it comes to our family, our choice to go wheat-free was based on the Biblical mandate to take care of the bodies God has given to us. As Christians, we know our bodies are temples of the Holy Spirit, so we should glorify God with our bodies (1 Cor. 6:19-20). Bodily training has value (2 Tim. 4:8). Just as we want our souls to be well, we should also pray to God for good physical health (3 John 1:2). Our choice to be wheat-free is motivated out of a desire for *good health*.

Just as we should never make an idol of food or any specific diet, neither should we ignore our diet. The body is not merely a temporary shell to be discarded or tossed aside. God is the creator of the body, and one day he will raise our bodies from death. We should love taking care of our bodies, because our bodies are a gift from God—an eternal gift.

MOVING FORWARD:

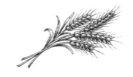

MAKING THE
WHEAT-FREE
TRANSITION

NO WHEAT?

WHAT IN THE WORLD DO I EAT?!

Where do I go now? What do I do? What do I eat for breakfast? No more bagels... cereal... toast... Danish? *No doughnuts!* And what about lunch? No sandwiches? And dinner? No dinner rolls or pasta?

Alright, take a deep breath. You can do this. If we can do it, so can you.

Do not replace wheat with empty calories and nutritionally deficient foods. We've often heard, "It's easier now than ever to eat wheat-free." Well, yes that's true, but what has happened is a lot of people are relying on gluten-free "junk food"—you know, the food that you see when you go to the "gluten-free" aisle of the grocery store. If you are doing this for your health, then you must replace the grains in your diet with nutrient-dense foods—*real foods.*

FATS

Increase your fat consumption. Focus on healthy fats and eat lots of them. It's a myth that fat makes you fat (see intoxicatedonlife. com/WOWresources for more information). Fat is an excellent source of fuel. It nourishes the body as well as the mind. When you don't get enough fat, it will rob your brain of the raw materials it needs to function. Diets high in saturated fat have been found to be effective in the treatment of epilepsy, Alzheimer's disease, Parkinson's disease, and in the prevention of stroke.

> *It's a myth that fat makes you fat. Fat is an excellent source of fuel.*

Be sure you are using natural, real fats. Avoid fats like margarine, vegetable shortening, canola oil, and corn oil. Fats like coconut oil, olive oil, butter from grass-fed cows, palm oil, and lard you've rendered yourself from healthy pastured pigs should be staples in your diet that you eat in abundance. If you're eating plenty of fats, this will go a long way in decreasing your cravings for grains and sugar.

FOCUS ON NATURAL FATS:

• **Butter** (Preferably grass-fed brands like Kerrygold)	• **Olive Oil** Don't use for cooking over high heat.
• **Lard from pastured pigs** You can easily do this yourself by purchasing the back fat from a local farmer.	• **Macadamia Nut Oil** Only use over low heat.
	• **Flaxseed Oil** Do not heat.
• **Tallow from grass-fed cows** You can also make this easily yourself by purchasing fat from a local farmer.	• **Coconut Oil**
	• **Palm Oil**
	Healthy Fats WON'T Make You Fat!

STAY AWAY FROM:

• **All trans-fats**	• **Soybean Oil**
• **Vegetable shortening**	• **Safflower Oil**
• **Margarine & other "buttery spreads"**	• **Sunflower Oil**
• **Canola Oil**	• **Partially Hydrogenated Oils**
• **Corn Oil**	• **Peanut Oil**
• **Vegetable Oil**	• **Grapeseed Oil**

PROTEIN

Include plenty of protein in your diet. Eggs, grass-fed beef, pastured pigs, and seafood are all fantastic sources of protein that your body can use. Purchase the highest quality protein you can afford. (Learn more about grass-fed beef and eggs from pastured hens at intoxicatedonlife.com/WOWresources)

In addition to your standard meats, we'd also urge you to include organ meats in your diet at least once or twice a week. Do you cringe at the thought of eating organ meats? I (Trisha), personally can't stand the sight or smell of the stuff (I'm worse than a kid). But when it comes to nutrient-dense foods, liver and other organ meats are powerhouses!

Organ meats are the most concentrated source of nutrients. Vitamins, minerals, healthy fats, and essential amino acids abound! Organ meats are some of the best fuel sources you can put in your body.

Liver has loads of B vitamins and is the highest source of the important vitamin B12 (By the way, B12 is only absorbed well by your body from animal products). Copper, riboflavin, vitamin A, vitamin D, zinc, iron, and selenium are all plentiful vitamin and minerals found in liver. You don't have to serve up platefuls of liver for dinner. A little bit goes a long way, just sneak some liver in with some ground beef. Nobody will know it's there unless you tell them!

VEGETABLES & FRUITS

Eat plenty of vegetables and eat fruits in moderation. Better yet, eat produce that is "in season" for your part of the world. Dark leafy greens, in particular, are packed with vitamins.

Don't forget to eat plenty of healthy fats with your veggies. Many vitamins, including A, D, E, and K that are found in your fruits and vegetables are *fat soluble.* If you are not getting adequate fat when you eat your vegetables, your body can't use them.

SUGAR

Cut the sugar. Really, cut the sugar. Sugar is difficult to get away from, but extremely detrimental to your health.

You may even need to decrease or eliminate natural sugars from fruits for a time. Many kids (and adults) are addicted to sugar, and it can be difficult to break the addiction while eating even natural sugars. Again, eating plenty of fat will help decrease your sugar withdrawal along with the withdrawal from grains.

BAKING

As you read this book, are you mourning the loss of freshly baked chocolate chip cookies and loaves of fluffy bread pulled from the oven? We understand. Truly we do. I (Trisha) love to bake. I made cakes, cookies, and other yummy treats from a very young age.

But going wheat-free doesn't mean you are going *treat-free*. It doesn't mean you have to give up baking. It just means, you have to be a bit more creative.

Thankfully, there are a number of easily available alternative flours on the market today. Our two favorites are coconut flour and almond flour. They don't work exactly the same as wheat flour, but they make some tasty treats—treats that our whole family enjoys.

Many gluten-free bakers also use potato, rice, corn, tapioca, sorghum, millet, and more. You won't find these ingredients in my recipes. You may be able to get a more "bread-like" consistency with some of these alternate flour, they are nutrient-poor and very high in starch.

We focus on foods that are nutrient-dense and taste good. This doesn't have to be an oxymoron. You can still pull freshly baked treats out of the oven for your kids after school, you just have to get creative and be willing to experiment with new recipes and ingredients you may not be familiar with.

ARM YOURSELF WITH GOOD BOOKS

These tips are really just scraping the surface of information on nutrition, but if you start with doing these things, you'll be off to a fantastic start.

There are lots of fantastic books out there on healthy eating and how to give up the grains in a good way. We didn't personally read any of these in their entirety or become an avid follower of them, but we've read enough of them to point you to them if you're looking for some good structure for your eating habits. Be sure to check out our Weeding Out Wheat Resources page (*intoxicatedonlife.com/WOWresources*) for some recommendations.

PREPARE YOUR PANTRY AND YOUR KIDS

Preparation can make or break your separation from wheat. If you're not prepared, then you're likely to fail. You've got to think this through.

We'd highly encourage you to include your spouse, kids, and anyone else living in your home on this journey. If you are truly convinced this is the healthiest way to eat, why wouldn't you want to put your kids on the path to health, too? Yes, if your kids are older, it can be difficult, and you might be met with resistance, but it's worth spending the time to get them on board. Be sure you explain to them why you're changing your family's diet—why the bread and beloved pizza are going in the trash.

You also need to prepare your pantry. Go through your pantry and trash any foods you shouldn't be eating. If it's unopened and non-perishable, a better option may be to donate it to a local food pantry. Preparing your pantry is the easy part, but it will make sticking with this new diet so much easier.

PLAN YOUR MEALS

Sit down and figure out some options for breakfasts, lunches, and dinners. Plan out a week of meals at a time.

Eating real, whole foods takes more time because it's not as easy as throwing a Pop Tart at your kid for breakfast. Taking the time to scramble some eggs or pre-cook bacon so it's ready to go in the mornings takes some forethought and extra time. But it's worth it.

Lunches at our house are often leftovers from dinners. But if you don't have leftovers, what is your plan? Keeping lettuce, hardboiled eggs, meat, homemade dressing, and cheese on hand is great for a tasty salad.

ARM YOURSELF WITH DELECTABLE TREATS

Before you take the plunge, it might be worth taking the time to experiment with some alternative recipes. There are some fantastic sugar-free and grain-free recipe blogs out in cyberspace (It won't hurt our feelings if you check out our recipes). Find the ones that appeal to you and have fun in the kitchen! Experiment with new ingredients and combinations you've never thought of before.

We have a list of cookbooks and blogs you may want to acquaint yourself with on our Weeding Out Wheat Resources page (*intoxicatedonlife.com/WOWresources*).

Don't forget to sign up to receive your complimentary Weeding out Wheat cookbook at *IntoxicatedOnLife.com/WOWcookbook*.

YOU CAN DO THIS

Nineteenth century humorist Henry Shaw once said, "Health is like money. We never have a true idea of its value until we lose it." Instead of waiting for something to go observably wrong

> *"Health is like money. We never have a true idea of its value until we lose it."*

with your health before you make the shift away from wheat, make the shift now. What you gain from it will be worth far more than what you lose.

RESOURCES
HELPFUL LINKS

WEEDING OUT WHEAT RESOURCES

This is a collection of links to cookbooks, blogs that feature healthy gluten-free recipes, and further educational materials to get you started. **Go to intoxicatedonlife.com/ WOWresources**

FREE WHEAT-FREE COOKBOOK

We're putting together a cookbook with some of our favorite wheat-free treats. Because you purchased this book, you're entitled to a free copy of the cookbook. **Sign up to receive your free copy intoxicatedonlife.com/WOWcookbook**

WEEDING OUT WHEAT FACEBOOK GROUP

Weeding Out Wheat Facebook Support Group: If you're looking for a community of individuals to connect with that will help you on your wheat-free journey, look no further. We've created a group for seasoned wheat-free vetrans and those who haven't even gotten started yet. This group will offer you encouragement, advice, recipes, and information. **Join us at facebook.com/groups/WeedingOutWheat**

Follow & Contact Links

- Facebook: facebook.com/intoxicatedonlife

- Twitter: twitter.com/intoxonlife

- Pinterest: pinterest.com/trishagrrl

- Email: IntoxicatedOnLifeMail@gmail.com

ENDNOTES

[1] Shewry PR. "Wheat." *Journal of Experimental Botany* 60, 2009 (6): 1537-1553.

[2] Gillis J. "Norman Borlaug, Plant Scientist Who Fought Famine, Dies at 95." *The New York Times*. 2009, Sept 13.

[3] "Norman Borlaug: The man who fed the world." *The Wall Street Journal*. 2009, Sept 13.

[4] Magaña-Gómez JA, de la Barca AM. "Risk assessment of genetically modified crops for nutrition and health." *Nutritional Reviews*. 2009 Jan 67(1): 1-16.

[5] Gao X, Liu SW, Sun Q, Xia GM. "High frequency of HMW-GS sequence variation through somatic hybridization between Agropyron elongatum and common wheat." *Planta*. 2010 Jan; 231(2): 245-250.

[6] van den Broeck HC, de Jong HC, Salentijn EM, Dekking L, Bosch D, Hamer RJ, Gilissen LJ, van der Meer IM, Smulders MJ. "Presence of celiac disease epitopes in modern and old hexaploid wheat varieties: wheat breeding may have contributed to increased prevalence of celiac disease." *Theoretical and Applied Genetics*. 2010 Nov; 121(8): 1527-1539.

[7] Shewry, P.R. "Wheat"

[8] "Wheat Flour." WhatsOnMyFood.org. <http://www.whatsonmyfood.org/food.jsp?food=WF> (accessed Sept 12, 2013.)

[9] Rahimi MM, Bahrani A. "Influence of Gamma Irradiation on Some Physiological Characteristics and Grain Protein in Wheat (Triticum aestivum L.)." *World Applied Sciences Journal*. 2001; 15(5): 654-659.

[10] Warchalewski JR, Pradzynska A, Gralik J, Nawrot J. "The effect of gamma and microwave irradiation of wheat grain on development parameters of some stored grain pests." *Nahrung*. 2000 Dec; 44(6): 411-414.

[11] Keener KM. "To Zap or not to Zap?" Department of Food Science Food Irradiation, NCSU. <http://www.ces.ncsu.edu/depts/foodsci/ext/pubs/irradiation.pdf> (accessed Sept 14, 2013.)

[12] Food irradiation Q&A's. (n.d.). Public Citizen., Center for Food Safety & Food & Water Watch. (2006). Food irradiation: A gross failure. Washington, DC: Jenkins & Worth.

[13] Raul F, Gossé F, Delincée H, Hartwig A, Marchioni E, Miesch M, Burnouf D. "Food-borne radiolytic compounds (2-alkylcyclobutanones) may promote experimental colon carcinogenesis." *Nutrition and Cancer*. 2002; 44(2): 188-191.

[14] Delincée H, Pool-Zobel, B. "Genotoxic properties of 2-dodecylcyclobutanone, a compound formed on irradiation of food containing fat." *Radiation Physics and Chemistry.* 1998; 52: 39-42.

[15] Public Citizen & GRACE. "Bad taste: The disturbing truth about the world health organization's endorsement of food irradiation." Washington, DC, & Global Resource Action Center for the Environment, New York, NY. 2002.

[16] "Potential Health Hazards of Food Irradiation: Verbatim Excerpts from Expert Testimony." U.S. Congressional Hearings into Food Irradiation. House Committee on Energy and Commerce, Subcommittee on Health and the Environment. 1987, June 19. <http://www.ccnr.org/food_irradiation.html> (accessed September 12, 2013.)

[17] "Broadbalk Winter Wheat Experiment." The Electronic Rothamsted Archive <http://www.era.rothamsted.ac.uk/index.php?area=home&page=index&dataset=4> (accessed Sept 13, 2013.)

[18] Fan MS, Zhao FJ, Fairweather-Tait SJ, Poulton PR, Dunham SJ, McGrath SP. "Evidence of decreasing mineral density in wheat grain over the last 160 years." *Journal of Trace Elements in Medicine and Biology.* 2008; 22(4): 315-324.

[19] Zhao FJ, Sua YH, Dunham SJ, Rakszegi M, Bedob Z, McGrath SP, Shewry PR. "Variation in mineral micronutrient concentrations in grain of wheat lines of diverse origin." *Journal of Cereal Science.* 2009 Mar; 49(2): 290–295

[20] Rubio-Tapia A, Kyle RA, Kaplan EL, Johnson DR, Page W, Erdtmann F, Brantner TL, Kim WR, Phelps TK, Lahr BD, Zinsmeister AR, Melton LJ 3rd, Murray JA. "Increased prevalence and mortality in undiagnosed celiac disease." *Gastroenterology.* 2009 Jul;137(1): 88-93.

[21] "Gluten Sensitivity on the Rise: A Real Problem or a Fad?" MyLifeStages.org. <https://www.mylifestages.org/health/gluten_sensitivity/gluten_sensitivity_on_the_rise.page> (accessed Sept 19, 2013.)

[22] Vehik K, Hamman RF, Lezotte D, Norris JM, Klingensmith G, Bloch C, Rewers M, Dabelea D. "Increasing incidence of type 1 diabetes in 0- to 17-year-old Colorado youth." *Diabetes Care.* 2007 Mar; 30(3): 503-509.

[23] Funda DP, Kaas A, Bock T, Tlaskalová-Hogenová H, Buschard K. "Gluten-free diet prevents diabetes in NOD mice." *Diabetes/Metabolism Research and Reviews.* 1999 Sep-Oct; 15(5): 323-327.

[24] Farrell R, Kelly CP. "Celiac Sprue." *The New England Journal of Medicine.* 2002 Jan; 346:180-188.

[25] Ji S. "Wheat: 200 Clinically Confirmed Reasons Not to Eat It." GreenMedInfo. com. 2012 Oct 7.

[26] Biesiekierski JR, Newnham ED, Irving PM, Barrett JS, Haines M, Doecke JD, Shepherd SJ, Muir JG, Gibson PR. "Gluten causes gastrointestinal symptoms in subjects without celiac disease: a double-blind placebo-controlled trial." *American Journal of Gastroenterology.* 2011 Mar; 106(3): 508-514.

[27] Tepper SJ. "A pivotal moment in 50 years of headache history: the first American Migraine Study." *Headache.* 2008 May;48(5):730-1; discussion 732.

[28] Dimitrova AK, Ungaro RC, Lebwohl B, Lewis SK, Tennyson CA, Green MW, Babyatsky MW, Green PH. "Prevalence of migraine in patients with celiac disease and inflammatory bowel disease." *Headache.* 2013 Feb; 53(2): 344-355.

[29] Cady RK, Farmer K, Dexter JK, Hall J. "The bowel and migraine: update on celiac disease and irritable bowel syndrome." *Current Pain and Headache Reports.* 2012 Jun; 16(3):278-286.

[30] Lionetti E, Francavilla R, Maiuri L, Ruggieri M, Spina M, Pavone P, Francavilla T, Magistà AM, Pavone L. "Headache in pediatric patients with celiac disease and its prevalence as a diagnostic clue." *Journal of Pediatric Gastroenterology and Nutrition.* 2009 Aug; 49(2):202-207.

[31] Hadjivassiliou M, Grünewald RA, Davies-Jones GAB. "Gluten sensitivity as a neurological illness." *Journal of Neurology, Neurosurgery, & Psychiatry.* 2002; 72:560-563.

[32] Ford RP. "The gluten syndrome: a neurological disease." *Medical Hypotheses.* 2009 Sep; 73(3):438-440.

[33] Freeman HJ. "Reproductive changes associated with celiac disease." *World Journal of Gastroenterology.* 2010 Dec 14; 16(46):5810-5814.

[34] Collin P, Vilska S, Heinonen PK, Hällström O, Pikkarainen P, "Infertility and coeliac disease." *Gut.* 1996 Sept; 39(3): 382-384.

[35] Farthing MJ, Edwards CR, Rees LH, Dawson AM. "Male gonadal function in coeliac disease: 1. Sexual dysfunction, infertility, and semen quality." *Gut.* 1982 Jul; 23(7):608-614.

[36] Choi JM, Lebwohl B, Wang J, Lee SK, Murray JA, Sauer MV, Green PHR, "Increased Prevalence of Celiac Disease in Patients with Unexplained Infertility in the United States: A Prospective Study." *Journal of Reproductive Medicine.* 2011 May-Jun; 56(5-6): 199–203.

[37] Hin H, Ford F. "Coeliac disease and infertility: making the connection and achieving a successful pregnancy." *Journal of Family Health Care.* 2002; 12(4):94-97.

[38] Stazi AV, Mantovani A. "A risk factor for female fertility and pregnancy: celiac disease." *Gynecological Endocrinology.* 2000 Dec; 14(6):454-63.

[39] Sher KS, Jayanthi V, Probert CS, Stewart CR, Mayberry JF. "Infertility, obstetric and gynaecological problems in coeliac sprue." *Digestive Diseases.* 1994 May-Jun; 12(3):186-190.

[40] Rostami K, Steegers EA, Wong WY, Braat DD, Steegers-Theunissen RP. "Coeliac disease and reproductive disorders: a neglected association." *European Journal of Obstetrics & Gynecology and Reproductive Biology.* 2001 Jun; 96(2):146-149.

[41] Pellicano R, Astegiano M, Bruno M, Fagoonee S, Rizzetto M. "Women and celiac disease: association with unexplained infertility." *Minerva Medica.* 2007 Jun; 98(3):217-219.

[42] Gasbarrini A, Torre ES, Trivellini C, De Carolis S, Caruso A, Gasbarrini G. "Recurrent spontaneous abortion and intrauterine fetal growth retardation as symptoms of coeliac disease." *The Lancet.* 2000 Jul 29; 356(9227): 399-400.

[43] Martinelli P, Troncone R, Paparo F, Torre P, Trapanese E, Fasano C, Lamberti A, Budillon G, Nardone G, Greco L. "Coeliac disease and unfavourable outcome of pregnancy." *Gut.* 2000 Mar; 46(3): 332-335.

[44] Stazi AV, et al.

[45] Pellicano R, Astegiano M, Bruno M, Fagoonee S, Rizzetto M. "Women and celiac disease: association with unexplained infertility." *Minerva Medica.* 2007 Jun;98(3):217-219.

[46] Ludvigsson JF, Reutfors J, Osby U, Ekbom A, Montgomery SM. "Celiac disease and risk of mood disorders—a general population-based cohort study." *Journal of Affective Disorders.* 2007 Apr; 99(1-3): 117-26.

[47] Poloni N, Vender S, Bolla E, Bortolaso P, Costantini C, Callegari C. "Gluten encephalopathy with psychiatric onset: case report." *Clinical Practice and Epidemiology in Mental Health.* 2009 Jun 26; 5:16.

[48] Ford RP. "The gluten syndrome."

[49] Pennesi CM, Klein LC. "Effectiveness of the gluten-free, casein-free diet for children diagnosed with autism spectrum disorder: Based on parental report." *Nutritional Neuroscience.* 2012 Mar; 15(2): 85-91.

[50] Whiteley P, Haracopos D, Knivsberg AM, Reichelt KL, Parlar S, Jacobsen J, Seim A, Pedersen L, Schondel M, Shattock P. "The ScanBrit randomised, controlled, single-blind study of a gluten- and casein-free dietary intervention for

children with autism spectrum disorders." *Nutritional Neuroscience*. 2010 Apr; 13(2): 87-100.

[51] Millward C, Ferriter M, Calver S, Connell-Jones G. "Gluten- and casein-free diets for autistic spectrum disorder." *Cochrane Database of Systematic Reviews*. 2004; (2): CD003498.

[52] Ford RP. "The gluten syndrome."

[53] Reichelt K, Ekrem J, Scott H. "Gluten, Milk Proteins and Autism: Dietary Intervention Effects on Behavior and Peptide Secretion." *Journal of Applied Nutrition*. 1990; 42(1): 1-11.

[54] Reichelt K, Knivsberg A. Lind G, Nodland M. "Probable etiology and Possible Treatment of Childhood Autism." *Brain Dysfunction*. 1991; 4: 308-319.

[55] Hoggan R. "Absolutisms Hidden Message for Medical Scientism." *Interchange*. 1997; 28(2/3): 183-189.

[56] Ludvigsson JF, et. al. "Celiac disease confers a 1.6-fold increased risk of asthma."

[57] "Wheat Allergy." Asthma and Allergy Foundation of America. <http://www.aafa.org/display.cfm?id=9&sub=20&cont=519> (accessed Sept 19, 2013.)

[58] I. Hafström, B. Ringertz, A. Spångberg, et. al. "A vegan diet free of gluten improves the signs and symptoms of rheumatoid arthritis: the effects on arthritis correlate with a reduction in antibodies to food antigens" *Rheumatology*. (2001) 40 (10):1175-1179.

[59] Uibo R, Panarina M, Teesalu K, Talja I, Sepp E, Utt M, Mikelsaar M, Heilman K, Uibo O, Vorobjova T. "Celiac disease in patients with type 1 diabetes: a condition with distinct changes in intestinal immunity?" *Cellular & Molecular Immunology*. 2011 Mar; 8(2): 150-156.

[60] Visser J, Rozing J, Sapone A, Lammers K, Fasano A. "Tight junctions, intestinal permeability, and autoimmunity: celiac disease and type 1 diabetes paradigms." *The Annals of New York Academy of Sciences*. 2009 May; 1165: 195-205.

[61] Bertini M, Sbarbati A, Valletta E, Pinelli L, Tato L. "Incomplete gastricmetaplasia in children with insulin-dependent diabetes mellitus and celiac disease. An ultrastructural study." *BMC Clinical Pathology*. 2001; 1(1): 2.

[62] Schuppan D, Hahn EG. "Celiac disease and its link to type 1 diabetes mellitus." *Journal of Pediatric Endocrinology & Metabolism*. 2001; 14 Suppl 1: 597-605.

[63] Holmes GK. "Coeliac disease and Type 1 diabetes mellitus—the case for screening." *Diabetic Medicine*. 2001 Mar; 18(3): 169-77.

[64] Saukkonen T, Vaisanen S, Akerblom HK, Savilahti E. "Coeliac disease in children and adolescents with type 1 diabetes: a study of growth, glycaemic control, and experiences of families." *Acta Paediatra*. 2002; 91(3): 297-302.

[65] Spiekerkoetter U, Seissler J, Wendel U. "General Screening for Celiac Disease is Advisable in Children with Type 1 Diabetes." *Hormone and Metabolic Research*. 2002 Apr; 34(4): 192-195.

[66] Barera G, Bonfanti R, Viscardi M, Bazzigaluppi E, Calori G, Meschi F, Bianchi C, Chiumello G. "Occurrence of celiac disease after onset of type 1 diabetes: a 6-year prospective longitudinal study." *Pediatrics*. 2002 May; 109(5): 833-838.

[67] Hansen D, Bennedbaek FN, Hansen LK, Hoier-Madsen M, Hegedu LS, Jacobsen BB, Husby S. "High prevalence of coeliac disease in Danish children with type I diabetes mellitus." *Acta Paediatra*. 2001 Nov; 90(11): 1238-1243.

[68] Aktay AN, Lee PC, Kumar V, Parton E, Wyatt DT, Werlin SL. "The prevalence and clinical characteristics of celiac disease in juvenile diabetes in Wisconsin." *Journal of Pediatric Gastroenterology and Nutrition*. 2001 Oct; 33(4): 462-465.

[69] MacFarlane AJ, Burghardt KM, Kelly J, Simell T, Simell O, Altosaar I, Scott FW. "A type 1 diabetes-related protein from wheat (triticum aestivum): cDNA clone of a wheat storage globulin, Glb1, linked to islet damage." *Journal of Biological Chemistry*. 2002 Oct; 278(1): 54-63.

[70] Scott FW, Rowsell P, Wang GS, Burghardt K, Kolb H, Flohe S. "Oral exposure to diabetes-promoting food or immunomodulators in neonates alters gut cytokines and diabetes." *Diabetes*. 2002 Jan; 51(1): 73-78.

[71] Scott FW, Cloutier HE, Kleemann R, Woerz-Pagenstert U, Rowsell P, Modler HW, Kolb H. "Potential mechanisms by which certain foods promote or inhibit the development of spontaneous diabetes in BB rats: dose, timing, early effect on islet area, and switch in infiltrate from Th1 to Th2 cells." *Diabetes*. 1997 Apr; 46(4): 589-598.

[72] Scott FW. "Food-induced type 1 diabetes in the BB Rat." *Diabetes/Metabolism Review*. 1996 Dec; 12(4): 341-359.

[73] Shor DB, Barzilai O, Ram M, Izhaky D, Porat-Katz BS, Chapman J, Blank M, Anaya JM, Shoenfeld Y. "Gluten sensitivity in multiple sclerosis: experimental myth or clinical truth?" *The Annals of New York Academy of Sciences*. 2009 Sep; 1173: 343-349.

[74] Cuoco L, Certo M, Jorizzo RA, De Vitis I, Tursi A, Papa A, De Marinis L, Fedeli P, Fedeli G, Gasbarrini G. "Prevalence and early diagnosis of coeliac disease in autoimmune thyroid disorders." *Italian Journal of Gastroenterology and Hepatology*. 1999 May; 31(4): 283-287.

[75] Akçay MN, Akçay G. "The presence of the antigliadin antibodies in autoimmune thyroid diseases." *Hepatogastroenterology.* 2003 Dec; 50 Suppl 2: cclxxix-cclxxx.

[76] Fasano A. "Leaky gut and autoimmune diseases." *Clinical Reviews in Allergy & Immunology.* 2012 Feb; 42(1): 71-78.

[77] Meadows, S. "The Boy with the Thorn in His Joints." New York Times, 2013, Feb. <http://www.nytimes.com/2013/02/03/magazine/the-boy-with-a-thorn-in-his-joints.html> (accessed September 19, 2013)

[78] Junker Y, Zeissig S, Kim SJ, Barisani D, Wieser H, Leffler DA, Zevallos V, Libermann TA, Dillon S, Freitag TL, Kelly CP, Schuppan D. "Wheat amylase trypsin inhibitors drive intestinal inflammation via activation of toll-like receptor 4." *Journal of Experimental Medicine.* 2012 Dec 17; 209(13): 2395-2408.

[79] de Punder K, Pruimboom L. "The Dietary Intake of Wheat and other Cereal Grains and Their Role in Inflammation." *Nutrients.* 2013; 5(3): 771-787

[80] Masters RC, Liese AD, Hanley AJ. "Whole and Refined Grain Intakes Are Related to Inflammatory Protein Concentrations in Human Plasma." *The Journal of Nutrition.* 2010 Mar; 140(3): 587-594.

[81] MacDonald TT, Monteleone G. "Immunity, Inflammation, and Allergy in Gut." *Science.* 2005 March 25; 307(5717): 1920-1925.

[82] Knip M. "Diet, Gut, and Type 1 Diabetes: Role of Wheat-Derived Peptides?" *Diabetes.* 2009 Aug; 58(8): 1723-1724.

[83] Bernardo D, Garrote JA, Arranz E. "Is gliadin really safe for non-coeliac individuals? Production of interleukin 15 in biopsy culture from non-coeliac individuals challenged with gliadin peptides." *Gut.* 2007 June; 58(6): 889-890.

[84] Biesiekierski JR, et al.

[85] Sapone A, Bai JC, Ciacci C, Dolinsek J, Green PH, Hadjivassiliou M, Kaukinen K, Rostami K, Sanders DS, Schumann M, Ullrich R, Villalta D, Volta U, Catassi C, Fasano A. "Spectrum of gluten-related disorders: consensus on new nomenclature and classification." *BMC Medicine.* 2012 Feb 7; 10:13.

[86] Drago S, El Asmar R, Di Pierro M, Grazia Clemente M, Tripathi A, Sapone A, Thakar M, Iacono G, Carroccio A, D'Agate C, Not T, Zampini L, Catassi C, Fasano A. "Gliadin, zonulin and gut permeability: Effects on celiac and non-celiac intestinal mucosa and intestinal cell lines." *Scandinavian Journal of Gastroenterology.* 2006 Apr; 41(4): 408-419.

[87] Bernardo D, et. al.

[88] Freed DLJ. "Do dietary lectins cause disease? The evidence is suggestive—and raises interesting possibilities for treatment." *British Medical Journal.* 1999 Apr 17; 318(7190): 1023-1024.

[89] Komath SS, Kavithab M, Swamy MJ. "Beyond carbohydrate binding: new directions in plant lectin research." *Organic & Biomolecular Chemistry.* 2006; 4: 973-988.

[90] Jönsson T, Olsson S, Ahrén B, Bøg-Hansen TV, Dole A, Lindeberg S. "Agrarian diet and diseases of affluence—Do evolutionary novel dietary lectins cause leptin resistance?" *BMC Endocrine Disorders.* 2005; 5:10.

[91] Sharon N, Lis H. "History of lectins: from hemagglutinins to biological recognition molecules." *Glycobiology.* 2004; 14(11): 53R-62R.

[92] Greger JL. "Nondigestible Carbohydrates and Mineral Bioavailability." *The Journal of Nutrition.* 1999 Jul 1; 129(7): 1434S-1435s.

[93] "Epidemiology of Dental Disease." Lecture Notes: Dental Anthropology, Human Variation, and Hominid Evolution. University of Illinois at Chicago. <http://www.uic.edu/classes/osci/osci590/11_1Epidemiology.htm> (accessed Sept 13, 2013.)

[94] Vucenik I, Shamsuddin AM. "Cancer Inhibition by Inositol Hexaphosphate (IP6) and Inositol: From Laboratory to Clinic." *Journal of Nutrition.* 2003 Nov 1; 133(11): 3778S-3784S.

[95] Grases F, March JG, Prieto RM, Simonet BM, Costa-Bauzá A, García-Raja A, Conte A. "Urinary phytate in calcium oxalate stone formers and healthy people— dietary effects on phytate excretion." *Scandinavian Journal of Urology and Nephrology.* 2000 Jun; 34(3): 162-164.

[96] de Punder K, et al.

[97] Pennington CL, Dufresne CP, Fanciulli G, Wood, TD. "Detection of Gluten Exorphin B4 and B5 in Human Blood by Liquid Chromatography-Mass Spectrometry/Mass Spectrometry." *The Open Spectroscopy Journal.* 2007; 1: 9-16.

[98] Zioudrou C, Streaty RA, Klee WA. "Opioid peptides derived from food proteins. The exorphins." *The Journal of Biological Chemistry.* 1979; 254: 2446-2449.

[99] Hyman M. "Three Hidden Ways Wheat Makes You Fat." HuffingtonPost.com. 2012 Feb 18. <http://www.huffingtonpost.com/dr-mark-hyman/wheat-gluten_b_1274872.html> (accessed Sept 11, 2013.)

[100] Perou R, Bitsko, RH, Blumberg SJ, Pastor P, Ghandour R, Gfroerer JC, Hedden SL, Crosby AE, Visser SN, Schieve LA, Parks SE, Hall JE, Brody D, Simile CM, Thompson WW, Baio J, Avenevoli S, Kogan MD, Huang LN." Mental Health Surveillance Among Children—United States, 2005-2011." Morbidity and Mortality Weekly Report (MMWR). Center for Disease Control. <http://www.

cdc.gov/mmwr/preview/mmwrhtml/su6202a1.htm?s_cid=su6202a1_w>
(accessed September 10, 2013).

[101] Dohan FC. "Wheat 'Consumption' and Hospital Admissions for Schizophrenia During World War II. A Preliminary Report." *The American Journal of Clinical Nutrition*. 1966 Jan; 18(1): 7-10.

[102] Haas, S. V. and Haas, M. P. Management of Celiac Disease. Philadelphia, 1951. J. B. Lippincott Co.; Bossak, E.T., Wang, C.I. and Adlersberg, D.I. Clinical aspects of malabsorption syndrome (idiopathic sprue). In: The Malabsorption Syndrome, New York, 1957. Grune & Stratton, Inc.

[103] Cascella NG, Kryszak D, Bhatti B, Gregory P, Kelly DL, McEvoy JP, Fasano A, Eaton WW. "Prevalence of celiac disease and gluten sensitivity in the United States clinical antipsychotic trials of intervention effectiveness study population." *Schizophrenia Bulletin*. 2011 Jan; 37(1): 94-100.

[104] Samaroo D, Dickerson F, Kasarda DD, Green PHR, Briani C, Yolken RH, Alaedini A. "Novel immune response to gluten in individuals with schizophrenia." *Schizophrenia Research*. 2010 May; 118(1-3): 248-255.

[105] Kalaydjian AE, Eaton W, Cascella N, Fasano A. "The gluten connection: the association between schizophrenia and celiac disease." *Acta Psychiatrica Scandinavica*. 2006 Feb; 113(2): 82-90.

[106] Dohan FC, Harper EH, Clark MH, Rodrigue RB, Zigas V. "Is schizophrenia rare if grain is rare?" *Biological Psychiatry*. 1984 Mar; 19(3): 385-399.

[107] Pennesi CM, et. al.

[108] Millward C, et al.

[109] Samaroo D, Dickerson F, Kasarda DD, Green PH, Briani C, Yolken RH, Alaedini A. "Novel immune response to gluten in individuals with schizophrenia." *Schizophrenia Research*. 2010 May; 118(1-3): 248-255.

[110] Ford RP. "The gluten syndrome."

[111] Kraft BD, Westman EC. "Schizophrenia, gluten, and low-carbohydrate, ketogenic diets: a case report and review of the literature." *Nutrition & Metabolism (London)*. 2009 Feb 26; 6:10.

[112] Foster-Powell K, Holt SHA, Brand-Miller JC. "International table of glycemic index and glycemic load values." *The American Journal of Clinical Nutrition*. 2002; 76(1): 5-56.

[113] CyrexLabs.com

[114] Greco L, Gobbetti M, Auricchio R, Di Mase R, Landolfo F, Paparo F, Di Cagno R, De Angelis M, Rizzello GC, Cassone A, Terrone G, Timpone L, D'Aniello M, Maglio M, Troncone R, Auricchio S. "Safety for Patients With Celiac Disease of Baked Goods Made of Wheat Flour Hydrolyzed During Food Processing." *Clinical Gastroenterology and Hepatology*. 2011 Jan; 9(1): 24-29.

[115] Di Cagno R, Barbato M, Di Camillo C, Rizzello CG, De Angelis M, Giuliani G, De Vincenzi M, Gobbetti M, Cucchiara S. "Gluten-free Sourdough Wheat Baked Goods Appear Safe for Young Celiac Patients: A Pilot Study." *Journal of Pediatric Gastroenterology & Nutrition*. 2010 Dec; 51(6): 777-783.

[116] Di Cagno R, De Angelis M, Gobbetti M. "Sourdough Bread Made from Wheat and Nontoxic Flours and Started with Selected Lactobacilli Is Tolerated in Celiac Sprue Patients." *Applied Environmental Microbiology*. 2004 Feb; 70(2): 1088-1096.

[117] There is no shortage of materials available trying to answer the question about the alcoholic content of wine in the Bible. Some take the position that anytime wine is praised in the Scriptures, it must be talking about the non-alcoholic variety (i.e. grape juice). I take serious issue with this for several reasons, but space doesn't permit me to go into it here. Instead, I'll refer my readers to the fine paper written by Kenneth Gentry, Jr., "The Bible and the Question of Alcoholic Beverages," Criswell Theological Review, 2008 Spring. In this article he sets out to prove, among other things, that the wine in the Bible was "a fermented quality, alcoholic-content, potentially inebriating beverage."

[118] Teyssen S, Lenzing T, González-Calero G, Korn A, Riepl RL, Singer MV. "Alcoholic beverages produced by alcoholic fermentation but not by distillation are powerful stimulants of gastric acid secretion in humans." *Gut*. 1997 Jan; 40(1): 49-56.

[119] Chari S, Teyssen S, Singer MV. "Alcohol and gastric acid secretion in humans." *Gut*. 1993 Jun; 34(6): 843-847.

[120] Pfeiffer A, Högl B, Kaess H. "Effect of ethanol and commonly ingested alcoholic beverages on gastric emptying and gastrointestinal transit." *The Clinical Investigator*. 1992; 70(6):, 487-491.

[121] Gaffney J. "Red Wine Helps Kick-Start Good Digestion. Portuguese study finds the beverage triggers chemical reactions inside the stomach." WineSpectator.com. 2009 Oct 14. <http://www.winespectator.com/webfeature/show/id/40985> (accessed Mar 3, 2013).

[122] "Clean and Unclean Animals." JewishEncyclopedia.com. <http://www.jewishencyclopedia.com/articles/4408-clean-and-unclean-animals> (accessed Sept 11, 2013).

[123] "Wild Flowers of Israel." WildFlowers.co. <http://www.wildflowers.co.il/english/poisonIndex.asp> (accessed Sept 11, 2013).

19210786R00080

Made in the USA
San Bernardino, CA
17 February 2015